NMR IN BIOLOGY AND MEDICINE

NMR in Biology and Medicine

Editors

Shu Chien, M.D., PH.D.

Professor of Physiology
Department of Physiology
    and Cellular Biophysics
College of Physicians and Surgeons
Columbia University
New York, New York

Chien Ho, PH.D.

Department of Biological
    Sciences
Carnegie-Mellon University
Pittsburgh, Pennsylvania

Raven Press ▪ New York

Raven Press, 1140 Avenue of the Americas, New York, New York
10036

Made in the United States of America

Library of Congress Cataloging-in-Publication Data

NMR in biology and medicine.

Proceedings of the Symposium on Nuclear Magnetic
Resonance in Biology and Medicine, held Dec. 1984
in Taipei, and sponsored by the Academia Sinica's
Institute of Biomedical Sciences and Central Laboratory
of Molecular Biology, and the National Science Council
of the Republic of China.
  Includes bibliographies and index.
  1. Nuclear magnetic resonance spectroscopy—
Congresses. 2. Magnetic resonance imaging—Congresses.
3. Biomolecules—Analysis—Congresses. I. Chien, Shu.
II. Ho, Chien, 1934-   . III. Symposium on Nuclear
Magnetic Resonance in Biology and Medicine (1984 :
Taipei, Taiwan) IV. Chung yang yen chiu yüan. Sheng wu
i hsüeh yen chiu so. V. Chung yang yen chiu yüan.
Fen tzu sheng wu hsüeh tsung ho yen chiu shih.
VI. Kuo chia k'o hsüeh wei yüan hui. [DNLM: 1. Nuclear
Magnetic Resonance—congresses. QU 25 N738]
QP519.9.N83N67   1986   574.19′285   86-13757
ISBN 0-88167-231-9

  The material contained in this volume was submitted as previously
unpublished material, except in the instances in which credit has
been given to the source from which some of the illustrative material
was derived.
  Papers or parts thereof have been used as camera-ready copy as
submitted by the authors whenever possible; when retyped they have
been edited by the editorial staff only to the extent considered necessary for the assistance of an international readership. The views expressed and the general style adopted remain, however, the responsibility
of the named authors. Great care has been taken to maintain the
accuracy of the information contained in this volume. However, Raven
Press cannot be held responsible for errors or for any consequences
arising from the use of the information contained herein.
  Materials appearing in this book prepared by individuals as part of
their official duties as U.S. Government employees are not covered
by the above-mentioned copyright.
  Authors were themselves responsible for obtaining the necessary
permission to reproduce copyright material from other sources.

iv

Preface

There have been rapid advances in the application of nuclear magnetic resonance (NMR) to the study of biology and medicine. This is an exciting field in which a modern physical technique is utilized to investigate noninvasively the structure and function of a wide range of biological systems, from molecules to membranes to cells to organs, in living animals and man.

In order to introduce state-of-the-art concepts and technology in NMR to scientists and students, the Preparatory Offices of two new units in Academia Sinica, i.e., the Institute of Biomedical Sciences and the Central Laboratory of Molecular Biology, and the National Science Council of Republic of China invited international experts in the field to hold a Symposium on NMR in Biology and Medicine in Taipei in December 1984. The invited speakers kindly agreed to follow up the Symposium with manuscripts written in 1985-1986, thus making possible the dissemination of valuable information to the scientific community at large through the publication of this book.

This volume, which brings together research from laboratories that are actively working at the forefront of NMR in biology and medicine, will be of interest to investigators in all biomedical disciplines, including biophysicists, biochemists, molecular biologists, cell biologists, physiologists, radiologists, and physicians and surgeons in various fields.

Shu Chien
Chien Ho

Acknowledgments

The successful holding of this Symposium on Nuclear Magnetic Resonance in Biology and Medicine and the publication of this volume of proceedings have been made possible by the support and efforts of many organizations and individuals. We would like to especially thank President Ta You Wu of Academia Sinica, Dr. Paul N. Yu, Chairman of the Planning Committee of the Institute of Biomedical Sciences, Dr. Paul O.P. Ts'o, Chairman of the Planning Committee of the Central Laboratory of Molecular Biology, and Chairman Li An Chen and Vice Chairman Tsou Shuen Liu of the National Science Council for their strong support and continuous encouragement. We want to express our appreciation to the Veterans General Hospital and its Superintendent Dr. Chih Shuen Tsou for co-sponsoring this symposium and providing us with magnificent meeting facilities. We are indebted to the Planning Committee for the Symposium chaired by Dr. Sung Mau Wang, and especially to the Executives of the Planning Committee, Drs. Choh Yung Chai, Ching Er Lin, Yao Huai Lin, Weichen Tien, and Peter S.H. Yeh, and the staff members. Their efficient, thoughtful and dedicated work, has made the symposium run so smoothly and the experience of the participants so enjoyable. We also wish to thank the members of the Scientific Program Committee, the Advisory Committee and the Supporting Committee for their valuable advice, counsel, support and encouragement.

We are most grateful to the world-renowned leaders in NMR research who came from Canada, the United Kingdom and the United States to give us the superb, authoritative and stimulating lectures on the cutting edge of NMR research in biology and medicine. We are very fortunate to have these truly outstanding scientists here to make this a world-class symposium.

The Pre-Symposium Course and the Workshops, which are not published in this book, contributed significantly to the success of the symposium by providing the introduction and preparation beforehand and the amplification and supplementation after each session. For this, we would like to express our gratitude to the five Chinese scientists who came back from the United States to render these important services: they are Dr. Lou-sing Kan, the course-workshop organizer, and Drs. Ching-Nien Chen, Tai-Huang Huang, Wen-kwei Wu and Ching Yao. We also wish to thank Drs. Sung Mau Wang and Wei Chuan Lin for organizing an interesting pre-symposium program on the present state of NMR research in Taiwan.

We would like to thank the session Chairmen who ran the program smoothly and facilitated the scientific exchange. We also appreciate the active participation by the audience at the Course, the Symposium and the Workshops. In addition to the scientific sessions inside the auditorium, we also had exhibits by several NMR manufacturers: Bruker, Varian and Elscint, and we would like to take this opportunity to acknowledge their valuable contributions.

We would like to thank Dr. George B. Schuessler for his help and advice in transcribing the word processor diskettes from different sources and to Ms. Ethel Goodrich, Ms. Michelline Faublas, Ms. Silvia Rofé and Ms. Franca Rofé for their help in the preparation of the manuscripts for publication.

Shu Chien
Chien Ho

Contents

Introductions

The phenomenon of NMR was discovered independently by two physicists, Felix Bloch of Stanford University and Edward M. Purcell of Harvard University, in 1946. Bloch and Purcell observed that transitions can be induced between magnetic spin energy levels of certain atomic nuclei in a magnetic field. The energy required to cause transitions between these Zeeman energy levels corresponds to frequencies in the radiofrequency range. Rapid progress in NMR was made during the first decade after its discovery. In recognition of this important discovery, Bloch and Purcell were awarded the Nobel Prize in Physics in 1952.

In the 1950s, chemists readily perceived the potential applications of NMR spectroscopy to the field of chemistry. Chemical shifts, spin-spin coupling, and relaxation processes were observed in the early 1950s. Since then, NMR has been recognized as one of the indispensable tools for chemists in elucidating structures and dynamics of molecules in both solution and solid states.

The promise of new applications for NMR has encouraged the development of better intrumentation. During the late 1960s, with the availability of super-conducting solenoids (which can produce higher magnetic field strengths than the conventional iron magnets), powerful microcomputers, and space-age electronics, biological applications of NMR have become feasible. In the 1970s, high-resolution NMR studies of proteins, nucleic acids, membranes, and other systems in both solution and solid states were carried out by biochemists, biophysicists, and molecular biologists, including several of our symposium speakers.

Throughout its history, NMR spectroscopy has been a truly dynamic field, with new advances following in rapid succession. The application of NMR to living systems, both by imaging and *in vivo* spectroscopic methods, is one of the most exciting developments in biomedical sciences during the past decade. Again, several of our symposium speakers are pioneers of this new field of biomedical NMR. NMR imaging provides anatomical information comparable to, and in many cases better than, that provided by X-ray computed tomography (CT). Unlike X-ray CT, NMR imaging does not use ionizing radiation, but rather makes use of an interaction among an applied magnetic field, radiowaves, and atomic nuclei. In the case of *in vivo* NMR spectroscopy, this methodology provides, for the first time, a direct, non-invasive monitor of biochemical events in selected regions of living cells, tissues, or organs of live animals or humans. There is little doubt that these complementary NMR methodologies are in the process of revolutionizing clinical diagnosis and treatments of diseases.

The principal mission of the Academia Sinica is to advance knowledge through research. We are very excited by the recent advances in biology and medicine. Our commitment to biology and medicine is best illustrated by the establishment of the Institute of Biomedical Sciences and the Central Laboratory for Molecular Biology. Some of our distinguished visitors had a chance to visit the sites of these two new units of the Academia Sinica These two new buildings, which are under construction and are in close proximity, are expected to be ready for occupancy in 1986. We are delighted that the Preparatory Offices of the Institute of Biomedical Sciences and the Central Laboratory for Molecular Biology are jointly organizing this timely Symposium on NMR in Biology and Medicine. We are most grateful to our symposium speakers who are willing to travel long distances to come to Taiwan to participate in this event. Our speakers come from Canada, the United Kingdom, and the United States of America and are pioneers and leaders in the field of NMR in biology and medicine. It is truly an international conference on NMR.

I wish to extend my gratitude and appreciation to the organizers of this symposium, in particular Dr. S. Chien and Dr. C. Ho, who have done an excellent job in suggesting the topics and speakers. The local organizers such as Dr. C. Y. Chai and Dr. Y. H. Lin of the Academia Sinica, Dr. W. Tien, Dr. S. M. Wang, and Dr. T. S. Liu of the National Science Council, Dr. C. E. Lin of National Taiwan University, and Dr. P. S. H. Yeh of the Veterans General Hospital, as well as their staffs, have done an outstanding job in making this conference possible. I am also very grateful to the five young scientists, who are the instructors for the Pre-Symposium NMR Course as well as the Symposium Workshop, for coming back to Taiwan to participate in these two important programs. Finally, I would like to extend my deepest appreciation to the Veterans General Hospital for hosting this conference with its outstanding conference facilities.

Ta You Wu
President, Academia Sinica
Taipei, Taiwan, R.O.C.

Since the first observation of the NMR phenomenon almost 40 years ago, the development of the application of NMR has been a vivid demonstration of how a fundamental phenomenon in physics could be developed into such a powerful instrumentation, so powerful that it has come far beyond the expectation of the original discoverers. The power and the versatility of such instruments could only be achieved by the continuous merging of the ideas and interests of scientists of different disciplines and the continuous introducing into it the most advanced technologies. It took almost fifteen years after the discovery of the phenomenon to develop the first commercial high-resolution NMR spectrometer. As more than often is the case, the immediate beneficiaries of discoveries in physics are the chemists. The availability of the first high-resolution NMR spectrometer almost immediately cast a revolutionary impact on the research of apparently every branch of chemistry. By being able to derive such informative parameters as chemical shift, coupling constant, resonance intensity and relaxation time, chemists have found the most effective and reliable means for the elucidation of molecular structure, which is so vital to chemical research. Besides, chemists have also found the use of this new technique in providing precious information on complex thermodynamic equilibria, kinetic parameters of molecular dynamics in solution, nuclear electron spin-spin interactions in paramagnetic species, and chemically-induced dynamic nuclear polarization, just to name a few.

The pulse technique and computer have made the FT NMR spectrometer available. This improvement enables chemists to work on samples in extremely minute amount and the nuclei of scarce abundance, e.g. ^{13}C, ^{15}N, ^{29}Si, etc. While techniques such as magic angle spinning has extended the domain of NMR into solid state, superconductor and cryogenic advances have made possible the high-power high-field NMR which has attracted the interest of researchers in life sciences who deal daily with molecules of much more complexity. Now we come to the age of *in vivo* NMR and NMR imaging, specially designed for biological research and medical application.

The National Science Council has financed the setting up of a 400 MHz NMR coupled with a 200 MHz magnet for solid samples in the Hsinchu Regional Instrument Center. Scientists in Taiwan need to know more about this state-of-the-art instrumentation in order to upgrade the quality of their research. Therefore, the purpose of this symposium is twofold: it is both academic and educational. I understand that the Organizing Committee has gone to great length and certainly done a superb job to gather so many most outstanding NMR specialists to participate in this symposium. For this reason, and as the co-sponsor of the symposium, NSC is most grateful for their effort. On behalf of Dr.. Li An Chen, I sincerely welcome all of you, from local and afar, and wish you all the successess at the symposium.

Tsou Shuen Liu
Vice Chairman, National Science Council
Taipei, Taiwan, R.O.C.

On behalf of the Institute of Biomedical Sciences, I would like to extend our warmest welcome and greetings. The Institute was established in 1981 under the auspices of Academia Sinica. Its aims are to promote, encourage, coordinate and support research in both clinical and basic areas of biomedical sciences in Taiwan. From the outset it was decided that the Institute should be mission oriented, with special emphasis on research and training in these major areas: cardiovascular disease, infectious disease (especially hepatitis) and cancer, which are very prevailing and the leading causes of death in Taiwan. Research programs, however, will not be limited to these three areas, and studies in fields such as neuroscience and lipid metabolism will also be encouraged. Sections will be organized to include molecular biology, system biology, and public health and preventive medicine. Research related to molecular biology will be carried out in close cooperation with the Central Laboratory for Molecular Biology, including disciplines such as virology, microbiology, biochemistry, immunology and genetics. System biology will include areas like pathology, physiology, and pharmacology. In public health and preventive medicine we will emphasize epidemiology and biostatistics. The building of the Institute is under construction and expected to be completed in early 1986. The building will be used primarily for basic research. Concurrently, three Clinical Research Centers have been established, one in each of the three major Medical Centers in Taipei, to facilitate clinical research in cardiovascular disease, infectious disease and cancer.

This Institute is very pleased to serve as one of the cosponsors of this symposium on NMR, as this cosponsorship fulfills one of our objectives, i.e., to bring new knowledge and technology in biological sciences to Taiwan. The program of this symposium is very impressive and covers topics extending from basic molecular research to clinical application. For basic research, NMR spectroscopy is used for the study of biochemical structure, metabolic and dynamic aspects of protein-lipid interactions, peptides, nucleic acid and blood. In clinical application, NMR imaging is a very powerful tool to detect and delineate abnormalities in organs such as the cardiovascular system and brain. It offers new parameters to characterize the tissues with greater specificity than computer tomography scan and radionuclide scintillography, but without the potential biological hazards associated with ionizing radiation.

We are very grateful to Drs. Chien Ho and Shu Chien in the United States and the members of the Planning Committee and the Committee on Scientific Programs in Taiwan for organizing such a superb symposium and inviting distinguished speakers to Taiwan for this meeting. I also wish to express our sincere thanks to the five Chinese scientists, who graduated from universities in Taiwan and received advanced training in the United States, for the excellent Pre-Symposium Workshop they gave. On behalf of the Institute of Biomedical Sciences, I would like to express our deep appreciation to all the distinguished speakers and faculty members for their participation and hope that they will have an enjoyable and pleasant stay in Taiwan.

Paul N. Yu
Chairman, Planning Committee,
Insitute of Biomedical Sciences,
Academia Sinica

On behalf of the Central Laboratory for Molecular Biology, I wish to welcome you here and to express my gratitude to the speakers who came to share with us your knowledge and contributions in this exciting field of NMR. Also, as a worker in the field of NMR and as a friend of many of you, I particularly feel grateful and happy to have you all here joining us. I am especially grateful to Professor Sunney Chan, who introduced the field of NMR to me and with whom I published my first NMR paper 23 years ago. The Institute of Biomedical Sciences and the Central Laboratory of Molecular Biology represent the realization of the idealism and dreams of many scientists, particularly those of Chinese origin, who would like to envision how biomedical research should be conducted in the 21st Century. We are gratified to visualize the rapid progress we have made in the building construction. The buildings of the Central Laboratory of Molecular Biology and the Institute of Biomedical Sciences are in close proximity, and they will be connected by a tunnel. Full collaboration of scientific efforts will be made by scientists of these two institutions.

We need to fill the building with people, plans and passion to conduct research. I am particularly grateful for the leadership and support given to us by the Past President Shih-liang Chien and the present President Ta You Wu of Academia Sinica, as well as the leadership and support given to us by the National Science Council. A combined effort and close collaboration by the Council and the Academy will lead the way for a new dawn in scientific research in Taiwan and Asia. Hopefully, we will set up a model for others to follow.

While the building construction and planning are still in progress, we already are introducing the best science to Taiwan. Six months ago in this very hall, the first collaborative effort of Academia Sinica and National Science Council took place in an important symposium entitled "Molecular Biology of Neoplasia," which was also well attended. Now six months later, we come to a second important collaborative effort between Academia Sinica and the National Science Council. Through particularly the efforts of the organizers Professor Chien Ho and Professor Shu Chien, this Symposium on "NMR in Biology and Medicine" was organized to bring this new field to this country. I wish also to thank the Workshop instructors who paved the way for the symposium with their Pre-Symposium Workshop education, and all the staff members of the Central Laboratory of Molecular Biology and the Institute of Biomedical Sciences, particularly Dr. C. Y. Chai, Dr. Y. H. Lin and their staff, all committee members, and the Veterans General Hospital, who prepared the ground work for this symposium.

Paul O.P. Ts'o
Chairman, Planning Committee
Central Laboratory of Molecular Biology,
Academia Sinica

CONTRIBUTORS

Ralph J. Alfidi
Department of Radiology
School of Medicine
Case-Western Reserve University
Cleveland, Ohio 44106

Utpal Banerjee
Division of Biology
California Institute of Technology
Pasadena, California 91125

Robert R. Birge
Department of Chemistry
Carnegie-Mellon University
Pittsburgh, Pennsylvania 15213

Myer Bloom
Department of Physics
University of British Columbia
Vancouver, BC, Canada V6T 2A6

Aksel A. Bothner-By
Department of Chemistry
Carnegie-Mellon University
Pittsburgh, Pennsylvania 15213

Neil I. Chafetz
Department of Radiology
University of California
San Francisco, California 94143

Sunney I. Chan
Arthur Amos Noyes Laboratory of
  Chemical Physics
California Institute of Technology
Pasadena, California 91125

Britton Chance
Department of Biochemistry/
  Biophysics
University of Pennsylvania
Philadelphia, Pennsylvania 19104

Shu Chien
Department of Physiology
  and Cellular Biophysics
College of Physicians and Surgeons
  of Columbia University
New York, New York 10032

Jacques M.L. Courtin
Department of Chemistry
University of Leiden
2300 RA Leiden, The Netherlands

M. Joan Dawson
Department of Physiology and
  Biophysics
University of Illinois Medical School
  at Urbana-Champaign
Urbana, Illinois 61801

Susan R. Dowd
Department of Biological Sciences
Carnegie-Mellon University
Pittsburgh, Pennsylvania 15213

Harry K. Genant
Departments of Radiology,
Medicine and Orthopaedic Surgery
University of California
San Francisco, California 94143

Thurman Gillespy, III
Department of Radiology
University of Florida
Teaching Hospital and Clinics
Gainesville, Florida 32610

Robert G. Griffin
Francis Bitter National Magnet
  Laboratory
Massachusetts Institute of
  Technology
Cambridge, Massachusetts 02139

Gerard S. Harbison
Department of Physiology and
  Biophysics
Harvard Medical School
Boston, Massachusestts 02115

Clyde A. Helms
Department of Radiology
University of California
San Francisco, California 94143

Judith Herzfeld
Department of Physiology and
  Biophysics
Harvard Medical School
Boston, Massachusetts 02115

Chien Ho
Department of Biological Studies
Carnegie-Mellon University
Pittsburgh, Pennsylvania 15213

Lou-sing Kan
Division of Biophysics
School of Hygiene and Public Health
Johns Hopkins University
Baltimore, Maryland 21205

Paul C. Lauterbur
Department of Medical Information
  Science and Chemistry
University of Illinois
Urbana, Illinois 61801

John S. Leigh, Jr.
Department of Biochemistry/
  Biophysics
University of Pennsylvania
Philadelphia, Pennsylvania 19104

Tsou Shuen Liu
National Science Council
Taipei, Taiwan 107, R.O.C.

Johan Lugtenburg
Department of Chemistry
University of Leiden
2300 RA Leiden, The Netherlands

Richard A. Mathies
Department of Chemistry
University of California
Berkeley, California 94720

Patrick P.J. Mulder
Department of Chemistry
University of Leiden
2300 RA Leiden, The Netherlands

Shoko Nioka
Department of Biochemistry/
  Biophysics
University of Pennsylvania
Philadelphia, Pennsylvania 19104

Johanes A. Pardoen
Department of Chemistry
University of Leiden
2300 RA Leiden, The Netherlands

E. Ann Pratt
Department of Biological Sciences
Carnegie-Mellon University
Pittsburgh, Pennsylvania 15213

George K. Radda
Department of Biochemistry
University of Oxford
Oxford OX1 3QU, UK.

Brian R. Reid
Departments of
Chemistry and Biochemistry
University of Washington
Seattle, Washington 98195

Michael L. Richardson
Department of Radiology
University of Washington
School of Medicine
Seattle, Washington 98195

James E. Roberts
Francis Bitter National Magnet
* Laboratory*
Massachusetts Institute of
* Technology*
Cambridge, Massachusetts 02139

Gordon S. Rule
Department of Biological Sciences
Carnegie-Mellon University
Pittsburgh, Pennsylvania 15213

Steven O. Smith
Department of Chemistry
University of California
Berkeley, California 94720;
Francis Bitter National Magnet
* Laboratory*
Massachusetts Institute of
* Technology*
Cambridge, Massachusetts 02139

Paul O.P. Tso
Division of Biophysics
School of Hygiene and Public Health
Johns Hopkins University
Baltimore, Maryland 21205

Chris Winkel
Department of Chemistry
University of Leiden
2300 RA Leiden, The Netherlands

Ta You Wu
Academia Sinica
Taipei, Taiwan 11529, R.O.C.

Paul N. Yu
Division of Cardiology
Department of Medicine
University of Rochester
School of Medicine and
* Dentistry*
Rochester, New York 14642

Raphael Zidovetzki
Arthur Amos Noyes Laboratory of
* Chemical Physics*
California Institute of Technology
Pasadena, California 91125

I. SOLID–STATE NMR STUDIES OF BIOLOGICAL SYSTEMS

NMR in Biology and Medicine,
edited by Shu Chien and Chien Ho.
Raven Press, New York © 1986.

NMR and Biochemical Studies of Protein–Lipid Interactions in Membranes

Chien Ho, Susan R. Dowd, Gordon S. Rule, and E. Ann Pratt

*Department of Biological Sciences, Carnegie—Mellon University,
Pittsburgh, Pennsylvania 15213*

INTRODUCTION

Bacterial membranes are being used in our laboratory for increasing our understanding of structure–function relationships in cell membranes. There are a number of advantages in using bacteria, particularly Escherichia coli. They are easy to grow, and powerful biochemical and genetic techniques are available for working with them. In bacteria, the cytoplasmic membrane is a very active part of the bacterial cell, carrying out respiratory functions and mediating the transport of substances into the cell. A simplified system for studying membrane functions of bacteria was developed by Kaback and co–workers some years ago (13,14). Basically, what they did was to osmotically shock E. coli cells. The cytoplasmic components leak out, then the membranes reseal. These membrane vesicles, without cytoplasmic contents, can continue to carry out respiratory and transport functions. We have chosen E. coli membrane vesicles as our starting point for studying structure–function relationships in membranes.

Nuclear magnetic resonance (NMR) spectroscopy is a useful technique for learning about interactions at the molecular level. Thus, we would like to see if we could learn something about membrane vesicles using NMR (see Reference 9 and the references therein).

^{31}P NMR STUDIES OF E. COLI MEMBRANE VESICLES

We have carried out a ^{31}P NMR study of E. coli membrane vesicles (11) using a special E. coli strain developed by Hong and co–workers. They have been able to construct an E. coli strain which contains the phosphoglycerate transport system from Salmonella typhimurium (17). One of the difficulties in studying very concentrated cell and vesicle suspensions is providing sufficient oxygen to the system. Vesicles of this strain have the advantage that they can carry on active transport without the presence of oxygen, using phosphoenolpyruvate (PEP) as the energy source. Figure 1A shows that in the absence of an energy source, the ^{31}P NMR spectrum of these vesicles is not very informative. Only an inorganic

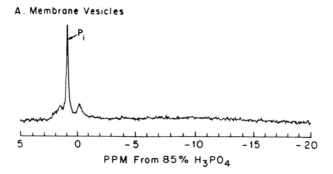

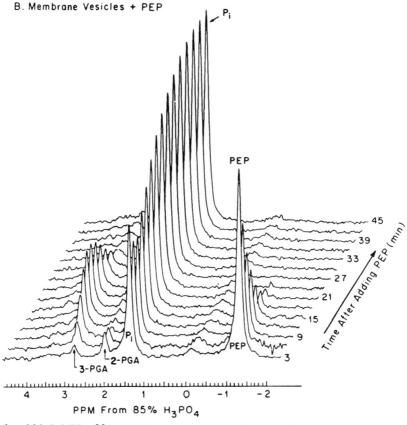

FIG. 1. 121.5 MHz ³¹P NMR investigation of the effect of phosphoenol-pyruvate on membrane vesicles from <u>E. coli</u> PSM116 containing a plasmid with the phosphoglycerate transport system from <u>S. typhimurium</u> (pJH7) at 30°C. A, membrane vesicles in the absence of PEP; B, membrane vesicles in the presence of 20 mM PEP. In B, the spectra, with the exception of the bottom one, are displaced slightly to the right to facilitate comparison. Taken from Figure 1 of (11), with permission. Note that the original assignments for 2– and 3–PGA as given in Reference 11 were inadvertently interchanged.

phosphate signal and a few sugar phosphate signals can be seen. However, upon addition of PEP, a number of interesting reactions occur (Figure 1B). A PEP signal appears, and there is an increase in the inorganic phosphate signal, due to the fact that in almost all the PEP solutions one prepares, there is a small amount of inorganic phosphate. But the most interesting part is the appearance of 2–PGA and 3–PGA signals. This would suggest that there must be enolase and also phosphoglycerate mutase present, otherwise we would not see 2– and 3–PGA signals. Enolase is inhibited by fluoride and if we add fluoride, we do not see the 2– and 3–PGA signals (data not shown). But we can still see the adenosine 5'–monophosphate (AMP), fructose 6–phosphate (F6P), and glucose 6–phosphate (G6P) signals. Adenosine 5'triphosphate (ATP) can also be observed, but the peaks are quite transient. To demonstrate the existence of ATPase, we have added N,N'–dicyclohexylcarbodiimide (DCCD), a powerful inhibitor of ATPase, to the vesicles (Figure 2). We can now readily see the α–, ß–, and γ–ATP signals, plus the AMP, F6P, and G6P signals. Thus, using NMR, we have demonstrated the existence in these <u>E. coli</u> membrane vesicles of enolase and phosphoglycerate mutase, and we have confirmed Hunt and Hong's finding (10) that pyruvate kinase is present, because we see ATP. We see AMP, so adenylate kinase must be present. We see the effect of DCCD on the utilization of PEP, so we know that Mg–ATPase is present. In conclusion, the <u>E. coli</u> membrane vesicles are enzymatically much more active than people thought a few years ago.

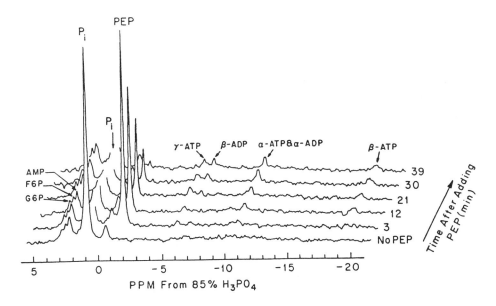

FIG. 2. 121.5 MHz ^{31}P NMR investigation of the effect of 100 μM N,N'–dicyclohexylcarbodiimide on the utilization of phosphoenolpyruvate by membrane vesicles from <u>E. coli</u> PSM116 containing a plasmid with the phosphoglycerate transport system from <u>S. typhimurium</u> (pJH7) at 30°C. The spectra, with the exception of the bottom one, are each displaced slightly to the right to facilitate comparison. The P_i peaks are omitted for clarity. Taken from Figure 3 of (11), with permission.

A bonus from our ^{31}P NMR study was learning something about intracellular and extracellular pH. When we look at the ^{31}P NMR spectrum of the E. coli membrane vesicles, we see only one signal for inorganic phosphate (Figure 3A). At the beginning, we were concerned that our spectrometer was not sensitive enough to see the inside and outside inorganic phosphate peaks. But we convinced ourselves that the sensitivity of our spectrometer was adequate by adding manganese ions. Mn^{2+} is a

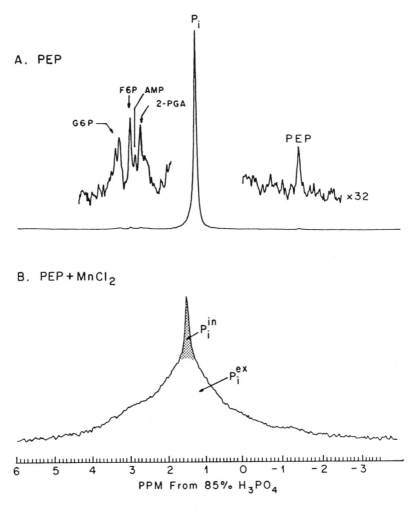

FIG. 3. 121.5 MHz ^{31}P NMR investigation of the effect of $MnCl_2$ on the ^{31}P resonance of inorganic phosphate from membrane vesicles of E. coli PSM116 containing a plasmid with the phosphoglycerate transport system from S. typhimurium (pJH7) at 30°C in the presence of phospho-enolpyruvate: A, in the absence of $MnCl_2$ (the inserted spectra are a 32-fold expansion); B, in the presence of 1 mM $MnCl_2$. Taken from Figure 4 of (11), with permission.

paramagnetic metal ion which can broaden the NMR signal. Upon the addition of Mn^{2+} to the vesicles, we see two signals, one very sharp, which is due to intracellular inorganic phosphate, and a broad component, which is due to extracellular inorganic phosphate (Figure 3B). Based on a pH calibration, we can conclude that within 0.2 pH unit, there is no difference between intra– and extracellular pH in this system.

STRATEGY FOR INVESTIGATING MEMBRANE INTERACTIONS

We have convinced ourselves that E. coli membrane vesicles are biologically very interesting, active and amenable to study by NMR, so now we want to carry out some studies on structure–function relationships in membranes. Membranes are made up of lipids and proteins. Thus, to understand how membranes carry out their function, we must learn about the nature of lipid–lipid, lipid–protein, and protein–protein interactions. In order to use NMR to study interactions in biological membranes, we need to fulfill the following requirements: (1) to select spectroscopic probes so as to derive molecular information; (ii) to develop techniques to label the membrane lipids and proteins with the spectroscopic probes; (iii) to find a system which can be reconstituted with spectroscopically–labeled components; and (iv) to obtain sufficient amounts of these labeled materials.

There are a number of different NMR techniques using different NMR–sensitive nuclei. The popular nuclei for studying protein–lipid interactions in membranes are ^1H, ^2H, ^{13}C, ^{19}F, and ^{31}P. They all have good points and bad points. They all can provide, in principle, both structural and dynamic information about the protein–lipid system. We would like to illustrate that ^{19}F is particularly useful as an NMR probe for studying interactions in membranes.

ADVANTAGES OF ^{19}F NMR FOR MEMBRANE STUDIES

There are a number of advantages in using ^{19}F in membrane studies. First, ^{19}F has a nuclear spin of 1/2 and a natural abundance of 100%. Second, ^{19}F has a high sensitivity, 83% that of ^1H. Third, there are no background resonances, because biological systems do not normally contain fluorine. Fourth, ^{19}F chemical shifts are 2–3 orders of magnitude greater than ^1H chemical shifts, and thus are very sensitive to environmental perturbations. And fifth, the large chemical shifts encountered in ^{19}F enable one to probe the motional states of the molecule not only through the averaging of magnetic dipole–dipole interactions, but also through the effect of motion on the anisotropy of ^{19}F chemical shifts. These five very good points warrant the use of ^{19}F in our membrane research.

^{19}F NMR STUDIES OF ^{19}F–LABELED PHOSPHOLIPIDS

We have carried out a systematic investigation using ^{19}F–labeled phospholipid (9). When dispersed above their phase transition temperature, phospholipids form multiple bilayer structures in water. Figure 4 shows a typical NMR spectrum of ^{19}F–labeled DMPC in water at 282.4 MHz. It is very broad. But if we can understand the line shape, we can derive valuable information about the structure and also about the dynamics of the lipid system. The only difference between normal DMPC and ^{19}F–labeled DMPC is the substitution of two fluorines for two hydrogen atoms in one of the chains. We would like to get some information from the fluorine atoms about the structural and motional properties of membranes. The line shape of the ^{19}F NMR spectrum in Figure 4 is due to the following types of interactions: the interaction between the two fluorine atoms, i.e., homonuclear fluorine–fluorine dipolar interaction; the heteronuclear proton–fluorine dipolar interaction; and the chemical shift anisotropy of the fluorine. One of our first hints for understanding the line shape came when we carried out a study of oriented bilayers of our ^{19}F–labeled DMPCs (Figure 5A) (3). When the angle between the normal to the bilayer and the magnetic field is 54.7°, the line shape is very sharp. The other angles show lines with a doublet. This is due to the two fluorine atoms, namely, the CF_2 group in the lipid system. When we carry out a study of non–oriented bilayers, the observed spectrum is a superposition of all different orientations (Figure 5B).

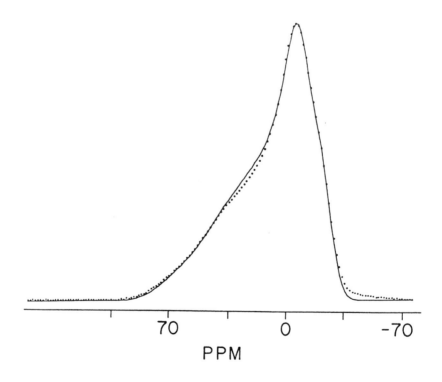

FIG. 4. 282.4 MHz ^{19}F NMR spectrum of 2–[8,8–[19]F$_2$]DMPC dispersed in D_2O (30/70, w/w) at 27°C: (........), experimental spectrum; and (———), computer–simulated spectrum. Taken from Figure 3 of (9), with permission.

A. Oriented Sample

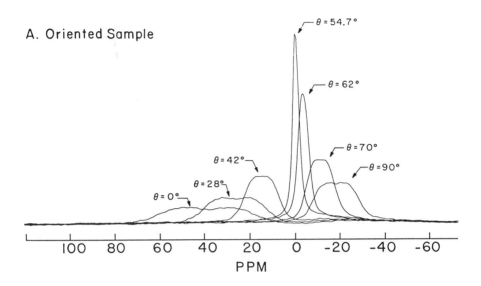

B. Non-Oriented Sample

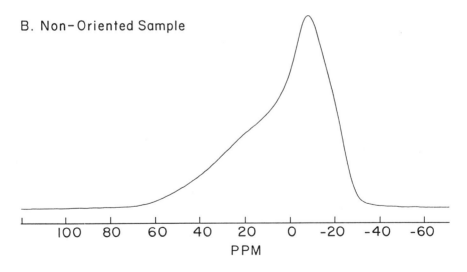

FIG. 5. 282.4 MHz ^{19}F NMR spectra of 2–[8,8–$^{19}F_2$]DMPC multilayers in H_2O at 27°C. A, spectra obtained for oriented lipid, aligned between glass coverslips, at θ = 0°, 28°, 42°, 54.7°, 62°, 70°, and 90°; and B, spectrum obtained for non–oriented dispersions of lipid. Taken from Figure 5 of (9), with permission.

Using this kind of analysis for oriented samples, we can derive some information about the chemical shift anisotropy, homonuclear dipolar interactions, and heteronuclear dipolar interactions. More recently, making use of a mathematical procedure, de–Paking, developed by Bloom and co–workers (26), we have been able to reconstruct spectra of oriented bilayers from spectra of non–oriented bilayers. We can see in Figure 4 that the experimental spectrum and the computer–simulated spectrum are essentially in agreement. This gives us a lot of confidence that our line–shape analysis is good. From the de–Paked spectrum, the separation of these two doublets is related to the order parameter, S_{FF}, which should tell us something about the time–average anisotropy or ordering of the F–F internuclear axis. By using this technique, we have been able to determine the order parameters of our lipid samples under different conditions. We can put the fluorine atoms at different positions along the acyl chains, and show that this gives different effects. We can show that the order parameter goes down as we increase the temperature (Figure 6). This is what we would expect, since at higher temperature there is more motion. To illustrate the sensitivity of ^{19}F NMR to the environment, we can change the water content. By reducing the water content, we increase the order parameter. Also by adding cholesterol, we increase the order parameter. These results are in good agreement with other published work using different techniques (12,18,24,27).

Even though our line–shape analysis gives us very good results, we would like to find another independent technique from which we can obtain the same kind of information as from the line–shape analysis. The spin Hamiltonian in the rotating frame for a lipid containing two fluorine nuclei and a large number of protons can be written as

$$\mathscr{H} = \mathscr{H}_{FF} + \mathscr{H}_{FH} + \mathscr{H}_{CSA}$$

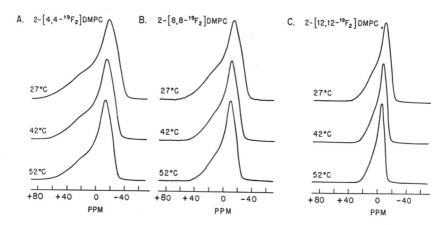

FIG. 6. 282.4 MHz ^{19}F NMR spectra of ^{19}F–labeled phospholipids dispersed in D_2O (30/70, w/w) as a function of temperature: A, 2-[4,4-$^{19}F_2$]DMPC; B, 2-[8,8-$^{19}F_2$]DMPC; and C, 2-[12,12-$^{19}F_2$]DMPC. Taken from Figure 2 of (2), with permission.

By using the Carr–Purcell–Meiboom–Gill (CPMG) pulse sequence, consisting of a 90° pulse, followed by a series of $180°_{90°}$ pulses, we can suppress both the heteronuclear H–F interactions and the chemical shift anisotropy. What is left is the homonuclear F–F interaction for the two fluorines. This is exactly what we observe, a nice Pake doublet (Figure 7). Thus, by using a suitable pulse technique, we can obtain the order parameter directly from the separation between the two peaks. A comparison of the order parameters that we have obtained from the line–shape analysis and from the multiple–pulse technique shows that they are in excellent agreement. This tells us that the ^{19}F NMR technique can really give us very informative results.

We would like to compare our results with other established techniques such as ^{2}H NMR. Oldfield and his colleagues (18) used ^{2}H NMR in a similar system with variously deuterated DMPCs. Figure 8 shows that the ^{19}F NMR and the ^{2}H NMR results for S_{FF} and S_{CD} are in very good agreement. The difference between them is no greater than 15%. In previous work, order parameters (S_{HH}) were determined from H–H dipolar interactions, and it was suggested that S_{HH} should be very close to S_{CD} (8) or about 10–15% lower than S_{CD} (19). So our ^{19}F results are, indeed, very good, and suggest that the perturbation introduced by the substitution of a CF_2 group for a CH_2 group cannot be very large. We are convinced that ^{19}F NMR can give the same kind of results as ^{2}H NMR. And there are several advantages in using ^{19}F NMR over ^{2}H NMR.

^{19}F NMR STUDIES OF BACTERIAL MEMBRANES

In the last section, we developed a technique to study lipid structure and dynamics in model systems. What we are interested in now is developing techniques to study labeled membranes in vesicles or the intact cell. We have synthesized a series of fluorinated fatty acids, 4–, 8–, and 12–difluoromyristic acids. We can incorporate these fluorine–labeled fatty acids into bacterial lipids by using fatty acid auxotrophs. These bacteria

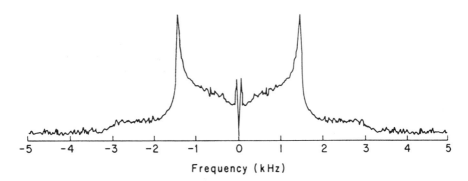

Frequency (kHz)

FIG. 7. 40 MHz dipolar ^{19}F NMR spectrum of 2-[8,8-[19]F$_2$]DMPC in 30% D$_2$O at 33.3°C, obtained with the CPMG pulse sequence $90°_y-(\tau-180°_{90°}-\tau)_n$: τ = 50 μsec; n=512; 90° pulse = 1 μsec; 1,000 scans. Taken from Figure 1 of (20), with permission.

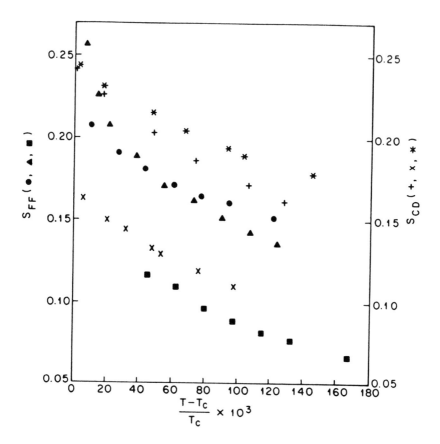

FIG. 8. A comparison of S_{FF} and S_{CD} of phospholipid dispersions as a function of reduced temperature: for S_{FF} data, ●, 2–[4,4–$^{19}F_2$] DMPC; ▲, 2–[8,8–$^{19}F_2$]DMPC; and ■, 2–[12,12–$^{19}F_2$]DMPC; and for S_{CD} data, *, 2–[4,4–$^{19}F_2$]DMPC; +, 2–[8,8–$^{19}F_2$]DMPC; and x, 2–[12,12–$^{19}F_2$]DMPC. The data for S_{CD} were taken from (18). Taken from Figure 3 of (2), with permission.

require unsaturated fatty acids for growth, and can incorporate 10–20% ^{19}F–labeled myristic acid into their lipids after one generation of growth. This is enough for our NMR studies. Figure 9 shows one of our first ^{19}F NMR spectra of intact cells obtained at 84.7 MHZ (7). Now we have convinced ourselves that by this approach we can incorporate fluorinated fatty acids into phospholipids of bacterial cells and obtain ^{19}F NMR spectra of membranes.

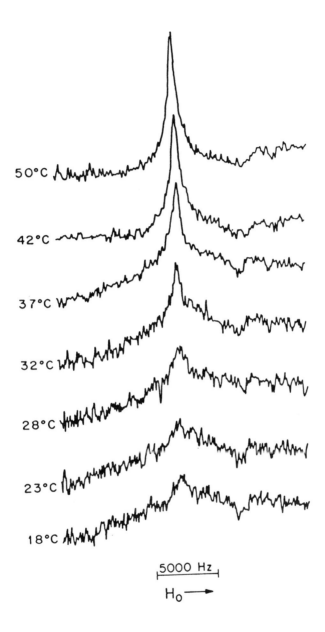

FIG. 9. 84.7 MHz ^{19}F NMR spectra of <u>E. coli</u> K1060B5 cells as a function of temperature. Cells were grown on 8,8–difluoromyristate at 37°C. Experimental conditions: sample concentration was 25 mg of protein/ml of D_2O containing 50 mM phosphate, 10 mM $MgSO_4$, and 50 μg chloramphenicol at pH 6.6. Each spectrum was accumulated over 10,000 scans. Taken from Figure 8 of (7), with permission.

D–LACTATE DEHYDROGENASE AS A MODEL FOR MEMBRANE
PROTEIN–LIPID INTERACTIONS

In order to study protein–lipid interactions, we also need to know something about proteins. We have to choose a membrane–bound protein or enzyme as the object of our study. Kaback and his colleagues (1, 15,25) and Futai (5,6) have shown that D–lactate dehydrogenase (D–LDH) is a very interesting membrane–bound enzyme of E. coli. It is involved in the respiratory chain and provides energy for transport of amino acids and sugars across the cytoplasmic membrane. It has a molecular weight of 65,000 and FAD is its cofactor. It requires lipids or lipid–like molecules for activity (4,16,28). Figure 10 is a schematic representation of a membrane vesicle, showing an enzyme, in our case D–LDH, in association with lipids and other proteins. A mutant strain has a defective protein (Figure 10B). In membrane vesicles prepared from this mutant, D–lactate cannot function as an electron donor for oxidase or transport activities. Purified D–LDH from the wild–type strain can be added to membrane vesicles prepared from the mutant and reconstitute oxidase and transport activities (Figure 10C). Thus, this system will allow us to put labels independently into either D–LDH or membrane lipids (Figure 10D). We have already demonstrated that we can incorporate ^{19}F into lipids and obtain useful information from spectra obtained from ^{19}F–labeled membranes. Similarly, we have used tryptophan auxotrophs of E. coli to incorporate ^{19}F–labeled tryptophan into proteins (21). We can then purify ^{19}F–labeled D–LDH and use it to reconstitute vesicles prepared from the D–LDH negative mutant (22).

Thus, we can label both lipid and protein with ^{19}F. Now we should be able to do some experiments. However, we still have one hurdle to overcome. NMR studies require a large amount of protein. The D–LDH protein in E. coli is normally present at approximately 1,000 copies per cell and contributes about 0.1% of the total cellular protein. Sixty liters of cell culture yield 3–4 mg of the enzyme, which is not enough for NMR studies. There are two general ways to increase the production of proteins in bacteria by recombinant DNA technology: (i) by cloning the gene of interest into extra–chromosomal plasmids with high copy number; and (ii) by increasing transcription of mRNA from the gene. We have used both methods (23). Using the clone of D–LDH isolated by Young (29), we have been able to construct a plasmid whose expression of D–LDH is under the control of the P_L promoter. When bacteria containing this plasmid are induced, we can get more than 300–fold overproduction. Induced cells average three times longer than normal cells, and about 30% of their total cellular protein is D–LDH. With this method, we can make enough D–LDH for NMR experiments.

With a cloned gene, we can also carry out DNA sequencing. We have determined the complete primary structure of 571 amino acid residues from the DNA sequence. We have also carried out an amino–terminal amino acid sequence determination and shown that our DNA sequence is in agreement with the amino acid sequence (23).

A. Hypothetical Bacterial Membrane Vesicle Containing Enzymes, Proteins and Lipids

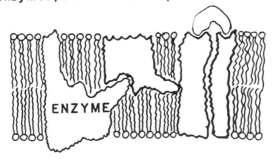

B. Membrane Vesicle from a Given Enzyme-Deficient Strain

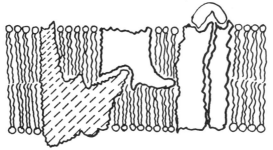

C. Membrane Vesicle Reconstituted with a Given Purified Enzyme

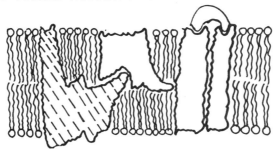

D. Reconstituted Membrane Vesicle with Spectroscopic Probes Incorporated into a Given Enzyme and Phospholipid

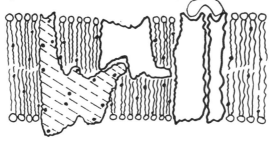

FIG. 10. Schematic representation of part of a membrane vesicle.

^{19}F NMR STUDIES OF 5F–TRP–LABELED D–LDH

The technique we have developed using ^{19}F labeling of protein is very general, and can be used with any amino acid, but in general, you do not want to label an amino acid which is present in large amounts, such as lysine or glutamic acid. You want to use one that is not present in such large amounts, so that you can see individual residues in the ^{19}F NMR spectra. Tryptophan is a very good example. From DNA sequencing, we found that there are five tryptophans in D–LDH, at positions 59, 384, 407, 469 and 567. Figure 11 shows the ^{19}F NMR spectrum of 0.2 mM 5F–tryptophan–labeled D–LDH in 1% Triton X–100 in the presence of 5 mM phosphate at pH 7.2 and 37°C. We see five signals. The fact that we see five resonances for five tryptophans tells us that each one has its own unique environment. Also, the line width of each of the five resonances is different, suggesting that there are differences in the motional properties among these five tryptophan residues. By observing these spectra under different conditions, we can obtain some very interesting information. If we change the lipid environment, resonances 2 and 3 shift, showing sensitivity to lipid environments. If we carry out a broad band proton irradiation and observe the ^{19}F resonances, we find that the resonances are reduced in intensity by different amounts. This suggests that the Trp residues have different levels of internal motion. To obtain more information about these residues, we carried out a solvent–induced isotope shift experiment with the enzyme. This can be done readily by changing the ratio between D_2O and H_2O. These experiments showed that resonance 4 is 60% exposed to the solvent and resonance 5 is 100% exposed to the solvent; it is on the surface of the molecule. This information is also consistent with our broad band ^{1}H decoupling experiment.

CONCLUSION

In conclusion, our experimental results have illustrated that by using NMR, genetics, and other biochemical and biophysical techniques, we can begin to study the nature of protein–lipid interactions in complex biological systems such as cell membranes. We believe that our model system, using E. coli membrane vesicles and the membrane–bound enzyme D–LDH, is a very promising one for obtaining information about structure–function relations in biological membranes.

ACKNOWLEDGMENT

Our membrane research is supported by research grants from the National Institutes of Health (GM–26874 and HL–24525) and the National Science Foundation (DMB 82–08829).

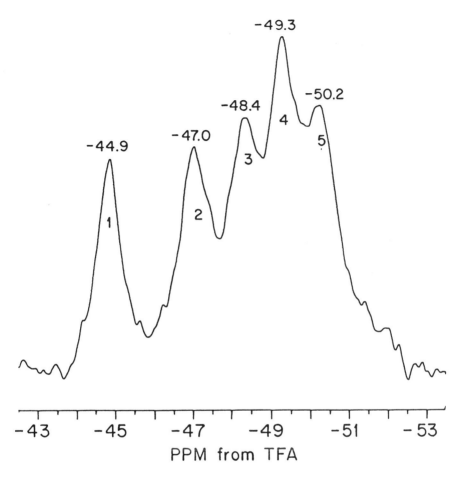

FIG. 11. 282.4 MHz ^{19}F NMR spectrum of 0.2 mM 5F–Trp–labeled D–LDH in 1% Triton X–100 in the presence of 5 mM phosphate at pH 7.2 and 37°C.

REFERENCES

1. Barnes, E.M., Jr. and Kaback, H.R. (1971): J. Biol. Chem. 246: 5518–5522.
2. Dowd, S.R., Simplaceanu, V., and Ho, C. (1984): Biochemistry 23: 6142–6146.
3. Engelsberg, M., Dowd, S.R., Simplaceanu, V., Cook, B.W., and Ho, C. (1982): Biochemistry 21:6985–6989.
4. Fung, L. W.–M., Pratt, E.A., and Ho, C. (1979): Biochemistry 18:317–324.
5. Futai, M. (1973): Biochemistry 12:2468–2474.
6. Futai, M. (1974): Biochemistry 13:2327–2333.
7. Gent, M.P.N. and Ho, C. (1978): Biochemistry 17:3023–3038.

8. Higgs, T.P. and Mackay, A.L. (1977): Chem. Phys. Lipids, 20: 105–144.
9. Ho, C., Dowd, S.R., and Post, J.F.M. (1985): Current Topics in Bioenergetics 14:53–95. Academic Press, New York.
10. Hunt, A.G. and Hong, J.-S. (1981): J. Biol. Chem. 256:11988–11991.
11. Hunt, A.G., Simplaceanu, V., Hong, J.-S., and Ho, C. (1983): Biochemistry 22:6130–6134.
12. Jacobs, R.E. and Oldfield, E. (1979): Biochemistry 18:3280–3285.
13. Kaback, H.R. (1971): Meth. Enzymol. 22:99–120.
14. Kaback, H.R. and Stadtman, E.R. (1966): Proc. Natl. Acad. Sci. U.S.A. 55:920–927.
15. Kohn, L.D. and Kaback, H.R. (1973): J. Biol. Chem. 248:7012–7017.
16. Kovatchev, S., Vaz, W.L.C., and Eibl, H. (1981): J. Biol. Chem. 256:10369–10374.
17. Masters, P.S. and Hong, J.-S. (1981): J. Bacteriol. 147:805–819.
18. Oldfield, E., Meadows, M., Rice, D., and Jacobs, R. (1978): Biochemistry 17:2727–2740.
19. Peterson, N.O. and Chan, S.I. (1977): Biochemistry 16:2657–2667.
20. Post, J.F.M., Cook, B.W., Dowd, S.R., Lowe, I.J., and Ho, C. (1984): Biochemistry 23:6138–6141.
21. Pratt, E.A. and Ho, C. (1975): Biochemistry 14:3035–3040.
22. Pratt, E.A., Jones, J.A., Cottam, P.F., Dowd, S.R., and Ho, C. (1983): Biochim. Biophys. Acta 729:167–175.
23. Rule, G.S., Pratt, E.A., Chin, C.C.Q., Wold, F., and Ho, C. (1985): J. Bacteriol. 161:1059–1068.
24. Shimshick, E.J. and McConnell, H.M. (1973): Biochem. Biophys. Res. Commun. 53:446–451.
25. Short, S.A., Kaback, H.R., and Kohn, L.D. (1974): Proc. Natl. Acad. Sci. U.S.A. 71:1461–1465.
26. Sternin, E., Bloom, M., and McKay, A.L. (1983): J. Magn. Reson. 55:274–282.
27. Stockton, G.W., Polnaszek, C.F., Tulloch, A.P., Hasan, F., and Smith, I.C.P. (1976): Biochemistry 15:954–966.
28. Tanaka, Y., Anraku, Y., and Futai, M. (1976): J. Biochem. 80: 821–830.
29. Young, I.G., Jaworowski, A., and Poulis, M. (1982): Biochemistry 21:2092–2095.

NMR in Biology and Medicine,
edited by Shu Chien and Chien Ho.
Raven Press, New York © 1986.

The Study of Lipid–Protein Interactions Using ^{2}H NMR

Myer Bloom

Department of Physics, University of British Columbia, Vancouver, BC, Canada V6T 2A6

INTRODUCTION

In this talk, I shall discuss the study of membranes using deuterium nuclear magnetic resonance (^{2}H NMR). It is appropriate to begin by explaining why the recent, impressive advances in the use of proton (^{1}H) high resolution NMR to determine the three–dimensional structure of small water soluble proteins are difficult to extend to the study of integral membrane proteins or other molecules in membranes.

Figure 1 provides a comparison of the ^{1}H NMR spectrum of a small water soluble protein (BPTI) in aqueous solution with that of rhodopsin in reconstituted membranes of dimyristoylphosphatidylcholine (DMPC) at a temperature above its gel–liquid crystalline phase transition (3). While BPTI exhibits a rich high resolution ^{1}H NMR spectrum with an enormous number of sharp lines visible over a range of a few kHz, the rhodopsin spectrum is broad and featureless, the high resolution spectrum being completely masked by proton–proton dipolar interactions. The dipolar broadening of BPTI, or any other small protein dissolved in water, is averaged out by its rapid, isotropic tumbling. However, the planar symmetry of the DMPC bilayer does not allow isotropic reorientation of solute molecules such as rhodopsin so that their residual dipolar interactions are usually much larger than the spread of frequencies associated with their high resolution spectra. As described by Dr. Robert Griffin in the next paper, it is now actually possible to answer certain types of well defined questions concerning the structure of an integral membrane protein such as rhodopsin by the use of sophisticated, high resolution, solid–state NMR methods. However, most NMR studies of membranes carried out up to the present time have involved broad line NMR methods using nuclear spin labels such as fluorine (^{19}F NMR), as described by Professor Chien Ho in the preceding paper, and deuterium (^{2}H NMR) which is the subject of my talk. After a brief introduction to the ^{2}H NMR technique and a review of some of the earlier, basic ^{2}H NMR studies of model membranes, I shall discuss two types of ^{2}H NMR experiments on lipid–protein interactions which were carried out in our laboratory. The

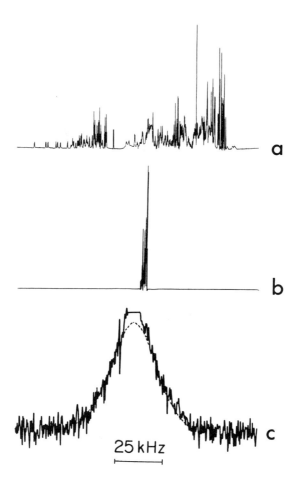

FIG. 1. Illustration of the different natures of the ^{1}H NMR spectra of proteins in water and in membranes. (a) The 400 MHz ^{1}H NMR spectrum of bovine pancreatic tryspin inhibitor, BPTI, in aqueous solution, exhibits a very rich high resolution spectrum with an enormous number of sharp lines visible over a range of a few kHz. (b) Spectrum of (a) on the scale of (c). (c) The ^{1}H NMR spectrum of rhodopsin reconstituted in model membranes of dimyristoylphosphatidylcholine with perdeuterated acyl chains (DMPC–d_{54}) exhibits a broad featureless line approximately 25 kHz wide (17). The high resolution lines are impossible to detect in this spectrum because they are masked by the relatively large proton–proton dipolar interactions, which are not averaged to zero by the slow anisotropic rotations of the protein in the membranes (Reference 3).

background material required to understand these experiments is available in review articles (3,6,9,10,14,18,20, 24,25).

REVIEW OF ²H NMR SPECTRA AND SEELIG'S WORK ON MODEL MEMBRANES

Deuterium labels can be introduced into molecules as a non–perturbing substitute for protons using chemical or biosynthetic methods. The main advantage in broad line NMR of ²H over ¹H is that ²H has spin one and hence three orientations as compared with two for ¹H; the coupling between the ²H quadrupole moment and the electric field gradient gives a basic spectrum which is a doublet having a splitting which is usually much greater than the dipolar broadening produced by neighboring nuclear spins. Measurement of the quadrupolar splitting provides similar but more easily interpretable information on local molecular structure and motion than is normally available from measurements of dipolar broadening of ¹H NMR spectra, although precise information can be obtained from the latter if sufficient care is exercised (17).

In the case of rigid C–²H bonds, i.e. those in acyl chains undergoing no conformational changes or rotations, the electric field gradient is (nearly) axially symmetric about the C–²H bond so that the quadrupolar splitting for an external magnetic field oriented at an angle θ with respect to the C–²H band direction is given by

$$\Delta v(\theta) \simeq (250 \text{ kHz}) \ [(3 \cos^2\theta - 1)/2] \qquad [1]$$

As illustrated in Figure 2a, the ²H NMR "powder spectrum" arising from a sample containing a superposition of randomly oriented C–²H bonds is spread over a range of 250 kHz but has a characteristic shape with two distinct peaks, the "Pake doublet", separated by $\Delta v(90°) \simeq 125$ kHz. These peaks correspond to the quadrupolar splitting at the most probable value of θ in a powder.

When rapid, axially symmetric molecular reorientation and conformational averaging of C–²H bonds takes place, the form of the powder spectrum is preserved but the overall width is reduced by a factor S = (1/2) <3cos²θ – 1>, where θ is the angle between the C–²H bond and the symmetry axis for the molecular motion. Figure 2b shows such a powder spectrum for S = 0.2. Thus the Pake doublet splitting of 125 S = 25 kHz in Fig. 2b is associated with membranes oriented such that the external magnetic field is parallel to the membrane surface, i.e. perpendicular to the symmetry axis for molecular motion, corresponding to θ = 90°.

Using the properties of the Pake doublet, Seelig and co–workers [see review articles (3,6,9,10,14,18,20,24,25), especially (24, 25)] determined the variation of the "orientational order parameter" S with depth in the liquid crystalline phase of model membranes, i.e. phospholipid bilayers containing no proteins. Effectively, Seelig measured the flexibility of acyl chains in membranes as a function of depth. He found a universal behavior of acyl chain flexibility corresponding to a roughly constant value of S ≃ 0.2 for that half of the acyl chain which is closer to the polar heads of the molecules at the membrane surface and falling to much smaller values in the membrane interior. Similar results had been found earlier in the lamellar phase of soap–water systems by Jean Charvolin (5). This important and fundamental work provided the motivation for subsequent theoretical studies of the nature of the gel–liquid crystalline phase transition. It also provided the basis for empirical investigations into lipid–protein interactions through their influence on the orientational order of the acyl chains of phospholipid molecules.

A simulated ^{2}H NMR spectrum of the type associated with hydrogen bonding in solids is given in Figure 3a. This spectrum has been simulated to match that part of the experimental spectrum (22) in crystalline samples of a synthetic α–helical polypeptide, lysine$_2$–glycine–leucine$_{24}$–lysine$_2$–ala-amide (K$_2$GL$_{24}$K$_2$A–amide), arising from the replacement of the protons in the N–H–––O hydrogen bonding sites by deuterons. The powder spectrum in Figure 3a is somewhat different from that of Figure 2a. The non–axial symmetry of the electron distribution about the N–H direction in the N–H–––O hydrogen bond gives rise to a non–axially symmetric electric field gradient of the ^{2}H nucleus (12,13) and is responsible for the form of the powder spectrum in Figure 3a. The spectrum of Figure 3b is that

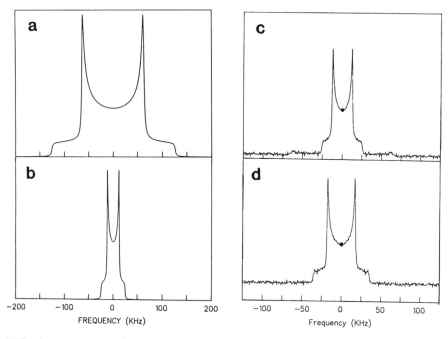

FIG. 2. Simulated ^{2}H NMR powder spectra arising from C–^{2}H bonds. (a) Top left: Spectrum of immobilized C–^{2}H bonds, i.e. S=1. (b) Bottom left: Spectrum representative of axially symmetric motional averaging of the C–^{2}H bond direction corresponding to S=0.2. (c) Top right: Spectrum corresponding to slow exchange on the ^{2}H NMR time scale between immobilized C–^{2}H sites (S=1) and sites having S=0.2. It has been assumed that 10 percent of the ^{2}H spins are on the immobilized sites. Noise has been added corresponding to a signal–to–noise ratio of 300 in the free induction signal. (d) Bottom right: Spectrum corresponding to the conditions of (c) in the fast exchange limit, i.e. S=0.28.

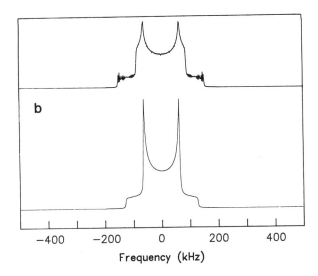

FIG. 3. (a) Top: Simulated ^{2}H NMR powder spectrum of the type associated with hydrogen bonding in solids. The spectrum is characterized by quadrupolar splitting parameters ($\omega_Q/2\pi$ = 150kHz, η = 0.16) associated with the crystalline form of the α–helical polypeptide, $K_2GL_{24}K_2A$–amide (22). The oscillations in the shoulders are artifacts of the spectral simulation and have no physical significance. (b) Bottom: Simulated ^{2}H NMR powder spectrum arising from the hydrogen bonding sites of an α–helical polypeptide rotating rapidly about its α–helical symmetry axis.

calculated for rapid reorientation of the N–H---O vectors in an α–helix about the symmetry axis of the α–helix (21). Note that the effect of rapid uniaxial rotation is to convert the powder spectrum of Figure 3a into a form identical to those of Figures 2a and 2b.

INFLUENCE OF LIPID–PROTEIN INTERACTIONS ON THE ^{2}H NMR SPECTRA OF THE PHOSPHOLIPID ACYL CHAINS

In order to appreciate the experimental strategy adopted by many workers in the investigation of lipid–protein interactions, look at the ^{2}H NMR spectrum in the liquid crystalline phase of an extremely simple model membrane (potassium palmitate–water mixtures) in which the acyl chains have been fully deuterated (Figure 4). The superposition of 31 ^{2}H NMR powder spectra illustrates Seelig's map of S versus position in the acyl chain or, equivalently, depth in the membrane. It is seen that the largest order parameters, corresponding to about S = 0.2, are obtained for the region of the acyl chain closest to the membrane surface.

It has been reasoned that since proteins are relatively rigid their introduction into phospholipid bilayer membranes should render the acyl chains of phospholipid molecules in their immediate vicinity more rigid

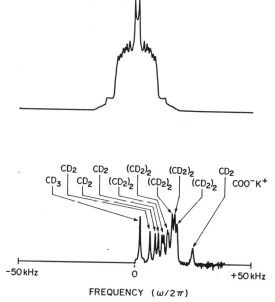

FIG. 4. Top: ^{2}H NMR powder spectrum of perdeuterated potassium palmitate at 65°C for a sample containing 50% potassium palmitate (by weight) and 50% H_2O. Bottom: Oriented spectrum derived from the above powder spectrum using the procedure of de–Pakeing of powder spectra (2,26). This spectrum is one side of a symmetric spectrum. The relationships between the peaks of the oriented spectrum and positions of the ^{2}H nuclei in the molecule are indicated schematically (Reference 2).

leading to relatively large values of S in ^{2}H NMR. Suppose that a fraction f of the lipids were in the immediate vicinity of the protein at any time with an order parameter S_p and the remaining fraction, 1–f, of the lipids had the original value S_o associated with the pure liquid crystal. Under these conditions, the nature of the ^{2}H NMR spectrum would depend on whether the rate of exchange between the two sites were slow or fast as compared with the frequency difference in the quadrupolar splittings associated with the two sites. These limits are often referred to as "slow or fast on the ^{2}H NMR time scale" of about 10^{-5}s. For <u>slow exchange</u>, two superimposed powder spectra characterized by S_p and S_o should be seen for each ^{2}H lipid site while <u>fast exchange</u> would give rise to one ^{2}H NMR powder spectrum characterized by a single average order parameter for each lipid site given by

$$S_{av.} = f\,S_p + (1-f)S_o$$

The types of spectra anticipated for $S_o = 0.2$, $S_p = 1$ and $f = 0.1$ for the slow and fast exchange limits are shown in Figures 2c and 2d, respectively.

It has been demonstrated that rigid molecules such as cholesterol (20,27) and the amphiphilic polypeptide $K_2GL_{24}K_2A$–amide (7) mentioned earlier produce perturbations to ^2H NMR powder spectra which are characteristic of the fast exchange limit (compare Figure 2b and 2d) when incorporated into liquid crystalline lipid bilayers. An example of the large influence of the polypeptide on potassium palmitate bilayers is shown in Figure 5 where it is seen that the addition of 1 molar percent of the polypeptide almost doubles the quadrupolar splittings of the potassium palmitate.

Searches have been carried out in several laboratories for ^2H NMR spectra characteristic of the slow exchange limit such as that shown in Figure 2c but no evidence has yet been found for lipid chains immobilized for times longer than 10^{-5} s by the presence of proteins in the liquid crystalline phases of phospholipid bilayer membranes. Furthermore, the average order parameters of the phospholipid acyl chains have been found to be essentially unchanged by the introduction of even large amounts of

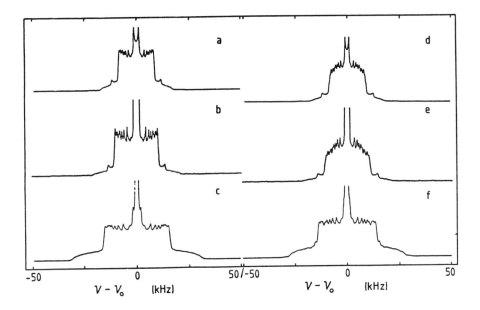

FIG. 5. ^2H NMR spectra of mixture of perdeuterated potassium palmitate and the polypeptide $K_2GL_{24}K_2A$ in 30% water by weight. The lipid–to–peptide molar ratios (L/P) and the temperatures used were: (a) L/P = ∞ (pure lipid) at 49°C; (b) L/P = 200 at 49°C; (c) L/P = 100 at 49°C; (d) L/P = ∞ at 65°C; (e) L/P = 200 at 65°C; (f) L/P = 100 at 65°C.

protein molecules. Most studies have not attempted to place an upper limit on the intensity of a hypothetical broad component in the wings of the observed crystalline ^{2}H NMR spectrum. With careful use of the Fourier transform quadrupolar echo method (6,8), however, it is possible to do a useful quantitative analysis of the hypothetical broad component, and this type of program was carried out in our laboratory in collaboration with P.F. Devaux and A. Bienvenue of the Institut de Biologie Physico–Chimique of U. of Paris on a sample of DMPC–d_{54} reconstituted with rhodopsin (1). In these experiments, all of the protons on the acyl chains were replaced by ^{2}H nuclei in order to increase the available signal from any hypothetical broad ^{2}H NMR spectrum associated with immobilized lipids. The spectra shown in Figure 6 for lipid/protein molar ratios of L/P = ∞ (i.e., pure lipid), 150, 50, 30 and 12 were all recorded above the temperature of the gel–liquid crystalline phase transition of the pure DMPC–d_{54} sample. As protein concentration was increased to a value L/P = 50, which is greater than the physiological concentration of rhodopsin in its native membrane, the individual ^{2}H NMR powder spectra were blurred but without a measureable increase in the average orientational order parameter (1). This is similar to results obtained in other membranes reconstituted with proteins (3,6,9,10,14,20,25). As described in the caption to Figure 6, the Fourier transform of the experimental spectrum of Figure 6c with its wings zeroed to eliminate any broad component, did not differ within experimental error from the quadrupolar echo used to produce the original spectrum (Figure 6f). In this manner, an upper limit of a few percent was obtained for the fraction of the acyl chains of the lipids immobolized by the rhodopsin in the sample (1) for times long on the ^{2}H NMR time scale.

Various conjectures have been advanced to explain the negative results described above. The proposal which I favor at the moment is that the ability of lipid bilayer systems to accommodate relatively large amounts of integral membrane proteins without much change in the average orientational order parameters of the lipid acyl chains is due to the matching of the hydrophobic thickness of the integral membrane proteins in natural proteins to that of the host phospholipids in order to minimize mechanical strain effects (19). Henderson and Unwin (11,28) have shown that integral membrane proteins consist of a set of predominantly hydrophobic α–helical elements which span the hydrophobic region of the lipid bilayers. In planning experiments on lipid–protein interactions, there has been a natural tendency to select combinations of phospholipid and protein molecules which could or do co–exist in natural membranes. Such a selection could maintain roughly the same geometrical constraints on the hydrophobic thicknesses of the lipid–protein mixtures studied as are present in the pure lipid systems. If the average value of the orientational order parameters reflects the membrane thickness, as it surely must to some extent, then the negative results of the experiments described above are easy to understand. In this context, the large increase in the order parameters of a soap bilayer due to the introduction of an amphiphilic polypeptide (Figure 5) and the relatively small perturbation of DPPC by the same peptide (7) is very striking since the equilibrium thickness of the pure soap bilayer is much smaller than that of DPPC.

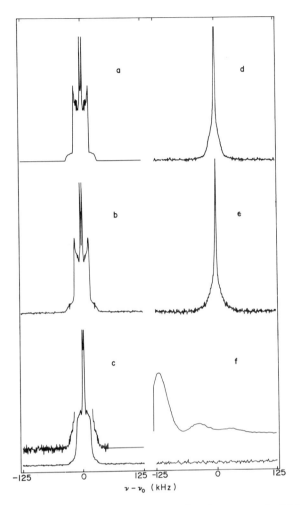

FIG. 6.   (a)–(e) are ^{2}H NMR spectra of mixtures of DMPC–d_{54} and rhodopsin for different values of molar lipid/protein ratio (L/P) at 23°C. The pure DMPC–d_{54} sample has its gel–liquid crystalline phase transition at 20°C. (a) L/P = ∞, i.e. pure DMPC–d_{54}; (b) L/P = 150; (c) L/P = 50; (d) L/P = 30; (e) L/P = 12. The individual powder patterns of the pure lipid in (a) are broadened with the addition of protein, (b) and (c), but the average quadrupolar splitting is unchanged. The spectra for L/P < 30 are different in shape but analysis shows that the average splitting is still unchanged. (f) The top trace shows the quadrupolar echo whose Fourier transform gave the spectrum of L/P = 50 in (c). The bottom trace shows the difference between this echo and that obtained from the Fourier transform of (c) with the wings of the spectrum zeroed as illustrated in the amplified spectrum shown in the top trace of (c). The fact that no residual difference signal was obtained in this manner, within experimental error, was used (1) to place an upper limit of a few percent of the number of lipids immobilized by the rhodopsin in this sample (Reference 1).

THE STUDY OF PEPTIDE AND PROTEIN MOTION USING ^{2}H NMR

Relatively little progress has been made thus far on the structure and motion of proteins in membranes. The first use of ^{2}H NMR to study integral membrane proteins directly was carried out recently using ^{2}H–labeled amino acids (15,16,23). These studies have given information on the dynamical properties of the side chains of integral membrane proteins. I would like to describe briefly an experiment carried out in our laboratory on the $K_2GL_{24}K_2A$–amide peptide incorporated into DPPC bilayers. This is a prototype experiment for the study of backbone motions of proteins in membranes.

In our experiment, the exchangeable hydrogens of the peptide were replaced by ^{2}H nuclei. Thus the ^{2}H were located at the N–H–––O hydrogen bonding sites of the α–helix and at the NH_3^+ positions of the lysines. The experiment was carried out using a lipid to peptide molar ratio of 50 to 1 mixed with ^2H_2O. As may be seen from the quadrupolar echo signal in Figure 7a, the ^{2}H NMR induction signal due to the heavy water was hundreds of times larger than that of the peptide deuterons. Indeed, the peak height of the Fourier transformed background ^{2}H NMR signal from the water was about 10^5 times larger than that of the much broader

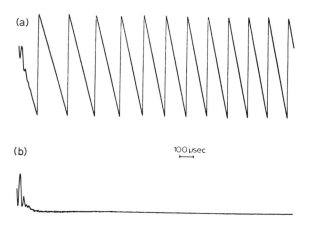

(a)

(b)   100 µsec

FIG. 7. (a) the ^{2}H NMR quadrupolar echo signal arising from a sample of DPPC and the polypeptide $K_2GL_{24}K_2A$–amide (L/P = 50) plus ^2H_2O (40% by weight) at 10°C. The peptide signal is seen only in the first 100 µs and is superimposed on the much larger and longer–lived ^2H_2O signal which overflows the computer memory 12 times during the 2048 µs shown in the figure. (b) The signal remaining after subtraction of an extrapolated polynomial fit to the data at times greater than 100 µs after the echo peak (4,22). The Fourier transform of this residual signal yields the spectrum of Figure 8a.

peptide signal. It proved to be essential to remove the enormous background signal from the quadrupolar echo induction signal, before Fourier transformation, using a subtraction method developed for this purpose (4,22).

The ^{2}H NMR spectrum from the sample in the gel phase of DPPC at 10°C as shown in Figure 8a. The broad feature of the spectrum is very similar to that of the simulated H–bonding solid state ^{2}H NMR signal shown in Figure 3a. Sitting on top of the H–bonding spectrum in Figure 8a is a narrower feature associated with the rotating $N^2H_3^+$ groups of the lysine residue. The observation of the characteristic H–bonding spectrum

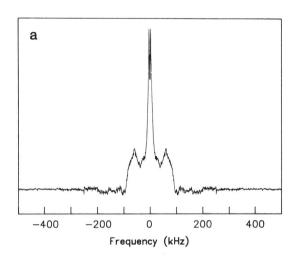

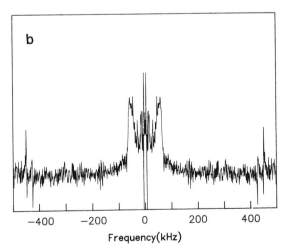

FIG. 8. (a) The ^{2}H NMR spectrum at 10°C of the hydrogen–exchanged polypeptide incorporated into DPPC as described in Figure 7. (b) The corresponding spectrum at 42°C.

demonstrates, as anticipated, that the peptide is unable to rotate rapidly in the gel phase of DPPC on the ^{2}H NMR time scale.

As the sample is warmed up from 10°C through the gel–liquid crystalline phase transition at about 40°C, it was observed (22) that the quadrupolar echo relaxation time, T_{2e}, decreased from its value of about 116 μs at 10°C through a deep minimum (<27 μs) to a value of about 100 μs in the liquid crystaline region. The minimum occurs when the correlation time, τ_c, for reorientation of the α–helical peptide about its long axis satisfies the condition $\Delta M_2 \tau_c^2 \simeq 1$, where ΔM_2 is the change in the apparent second moment of the ^{2}H NMR spectrum as a result of motional averaging when $\Delta M_2 \tau_c^2 \ll 1$. This short correlation time limiting behavior occurs in the liquid crystalline region as may be seen by comparing the spectrum of Figure 8b with the simulated spectrum of Figure 3b. Using the experimental values of ΔM_2 and T_{2e}, the geometry of the peptide and the theory of motional narrowing, it has been shown that the effective viscosity of the membrane is 1.1 poise (22), a value in excellent agreement with that obtained from fluorescence depolarization of proteins in DPPC bilayers.

These measurements demonstrate that it is possible to obtain information on the structure and motion of the backbones of integral membrane peptide and protein molecules. As an example, an interesting motionally averaged ^{2}H NMR spectrum was obtained in our laboratory recently (K.P. Datema and K.P. Pauls, unpublished) for Gramicidin A in the liquid crystalline phase of DPPC showing several inequivalent H–bonding sites in that ion carrier peptide.

ACKNOWLEGEMENT

I wish to thank Dr. A.L. MacKay for his helpful comments.

REFERENCES

1. Bienvenue, A., Bloom, M., Davis, J.H., and Devaux, P.F. (1982): J. Biol. Chem. 257:3032–3038.
2. Bloom, M., Davis, J.H., and MacKay, A.L. (1981): Chem. Phys. Lett. 80:198–202.
3. Bloom, M. and Smith, I.C.P. (1985): In: Progress in Protein–Lipid Interactions, edited by A. Watts and J.J.H.H.M. de Pont, pp. 61–88. Elsevier, Amsterdam.
4. Callaghan, P.T., MacKay, A.L., Pauls, K.P., Soderman, O., and Bloom, M. (1984): J. Magn. Reson. 56:101–109.
5. Charvolin, J., Manneville, P., and Deloche, B. (1973): Chem. Phys. Lett. 23:345–348.
6. Davis, J.H. (1983): Biochim. Biophys. Acta 737:117–171.
7. Davis, J.H., Clare, D.M., Hodges, R.S., and Bloom, M. (1983): Biochemistry 22:5298–5305.
8. Davis, J.H., Jeffrey, K.R., Bloom, M., Valic, M.I., and Higgs, T.P. (1976): Chem. Phys. Lett. 42:390–394.
9. Devaux, P.F. (1983): In: Biological Magnetic Resonance, edited by L.J. Berliner and J. Reuben, pp. 183–299. Plenum Press, New York.

10. Griffin, R.G. (1981): Meth. Enzymol. 72:108–174.
11. Henderson, R. (1981): In: Membranes and Intercellular Communications, edited by R. Balian, M. Chabre, and P.F. Devaux, pp. 229–249. Elsevier/North Holland, Amsterdam.
12. Hunt, M.J. and MacKay, A.L. (1974): J. Mag. Reson. 15:402–414.
13. Hunt, M.J. and MacKay, A.L. (1976): J. Magn. Reson. 22:295–301.
14. Jacobs, R.E. and Oldfield, E. (1981): Progr. NMR Spectr. 14:113–136.
15. Keniry, M.A., Gutowsky, H.S., and Oldfield, E. (1984): Nature 307:383–386.
16. Kinsey, R.A., Kintenar, A., Tsai, M.-D., Smith, R.L., James, N., and Oldfield, E. (1981): J. Biol. Chem. 256:4146–4149.
17. MacKay, A.L. (1981): Biophys. J. 35:301–313.
18. Mantsch, H.H., Saito, H., and Smith, I.C.P. (1977): Progr. NMR Spectr. 11:211–272.
19. Mouritsen, O.G. and Bloom, M. (1984): Biophys. J. 46:141–153.
20. Oldfield, E. (1982): In: Membranes and Transport, edited by E.N. Martinosi, pp. 115–123, Plenum Press, New York.
21. Pauling, L. and Corey, R.B. (1951): Proc. Nat. Acad. Sci. U.S.A. 37:241–250.
22. Pauls, K.P., MacKay, A.L., Soderman, O., Bloom, M., Taneja, A.K., and Hodges, R.S. (1985): Eur. Biophys. J. 12:1–11.
23. Rice, D.M., Blume, A., Herzfeld, J., Wittebort, R.J., Huang, T.H., Das Gupta, S.K., and Griffin, R.G. (1981): In: Biomolecular Stereodynamics, edited by R.H. Sarma, pp. 255–270. Adenine Press.
24. Seelig, J. (1977): Quart. Rev. Biophys. 10:353–418.
25. Seelig, J. and Seelig, A. (1980): Quart. Rev. Biophys. 13:191–261.
26. Sternin, E., Bloom, M., and MacKay, A.L. (1983): J. Magn. Reson. 55:274–282.
27. Stockton, G.W. and Smith, I.C.P. (1976): Chem. Phys. Lipids 17:251–263.
28. Unwin, P.N.T. and Henderson, R. (1984): Sci. Am. 250:78–94.

NMR in Biology and Medicine,
edited by Shu Chien and Chien Ho.
Raven Press, New York © 1986.

Solid State ^{13}C – and ^{15}N – NMR Investigations of The Retinal Protonated Schiff–Base Chromophore in Bacteriorhodopsin

G.S. Harbison *, S.O. Smith **,†, J.E. Roberts †, J.A. Pardoen §,
P.P.J. Mulder §, C. Winkel §, J.M.L. Courtin §, R.A. Mathies **,
J. Lugtenburg §, J. Herzfeld *, and R.G. Griffin †

*Department of Physiology and Biophysics, Harvard Medical School,
Boston, Massachusetts 02115; ** Department of Chemistry, University of California,
Berkeley, California 94720; † Francis Bitter National Magnet Laboratory,
Massachusetts Institute of Technology, Cambridge, Massachusetts 02139;
§ Department of Chemistry, University of Leiden, 2300 RA Leiden, The Netherlands*

INTRODUCTION

Bacteriorhodopsin (bR) is the single protein in the purple membrane of Halobacterium halobium (21). The protein has a molecular weight of about 26,000 and contains 248 amino acids. Its function is to pump protons across the membrane in response to the absorption of light, the resulting pH gradient being used in ATP synthesis. The mechanism of this proton pump has been of considerable interest over the last few years and has been studied with a variety of spectroscopic techniques (3,4,16,20). It is generally agreed that the pump has two parts — a proton wire and a photo–activated switch. The proton wire portion is thought to consist of a hydrogen–bonded chain involving the –OH groups of tyrosine, serine and threonine, the NH function of arginine, and the carboxyl groups of aspartic and glutamic acid. The switch portion of the pump consists of a retinal protonated Schiff base (PSB) which photoisomerizes from all–trans to 13–cis with an H$^+$ ion moving onto the wire. In this paper we discuss solid state NMR studies of certain aspects of the switch mechanism — i.e. the conformation of the protein–bound retinal.

RESULTS

bR occurs in trimers and these, in turn, form large patches of purple membrane. Because of their size (~50–60 Å thick, 0.5–1 μm in diameter) the patches tumble slowly and do not yield high resolution spectra with "solution NMR" techniques. Furthermore, attempts to solubilize the protein in detergents have inevitably led to problems with retinal stability and NMR spectra of poor quality (12,23). For these reasons solid state techniques are the methods of choice for obtaining NMR spectra of bR. In particular, we have used magic angle sample spinning (MASS) techniques together with specific ^{13}C and ^{15}N isotopic labeling (2,3,4). In addition to providing a means to observe a high quality spectra, the MASS NMR techniques also provide a considerable amount of other information. Spectra obtained in the slow spinning regime contain rotational sidebands which yield information on the chemical shift anisotropy. The conventional wisdom is that these sidebands are a nuisance and only make interpretation of the spectrum difficult. We will see below that the information they provide on chemical shift tensors is invaluable in interpreting the bR ^{13}C spectra.

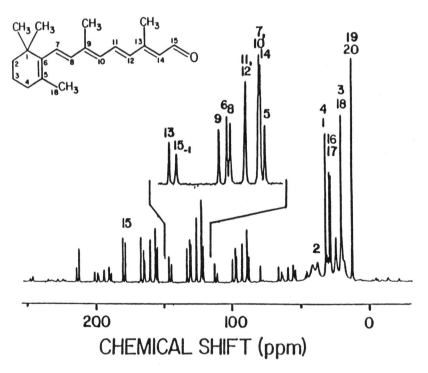

FIG. 1. ^{13}C MASS NMR spectrum of all-<u>trans</u> retinal spinning at 2.8 kHz. ν_{13C} = 79 MHz. The numbers correspond to the positions in the retinal molecule. The centerband region from the olefinic carbons is shown on an expanded scale in the inset.

A typical result illustrating the presence of rotational side–bands is shown in Figure 1, which is a MASS NMR spectrum obtained from all–<u>trans</u> retinal spinning at 2.8 kHz. The lines are numbered according to their assignments and the centerband portion of the spectrum is expanded and shown in the inset. In order to obtain accurate information on the anisotropies it is necessary to have strong sidebands present such as is shown in Figure 1. Typically, we then employ the computer fitting method outlined by Herzfeld and Berger (8) to obtain the anisotropies.

Figure 2 illustrates that high quality MASS spectra can also be obtained from hydrated purple membrane. In this case, we show a spectrum of bacteriorhodopsin into which ^{13}C–5–labeled retinal has been incorporated as described elsewhere (5). The right side of the spectrum is due to the aliphatic and methyl carbons and because their tensors are small, there are no sidebands associated with these lines. The prominent broad line at ~175 ppm is the C=O centerband from the 248 backbone carbonyls in the protein. Carbonyl sidebands are apparent on each side of the centerband, spaced at the spinning frequency. The arrowed line at 145 ppm is the centerband due to the ^{13}C–5 label in the retinal, and its sidebands from

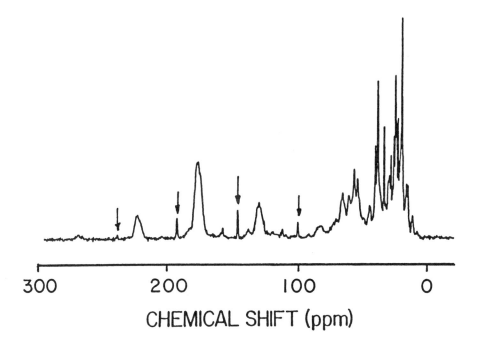

CHEMICAL SHIFT (ppm)

FIG. 2. ^{13}C MASS NMR spectrum of fully hydrated ^{13}C–5–retinal–bR. The arrowed line at 145 ppm is the centerband from the retinal. Its sidebands are also marked with arrows.

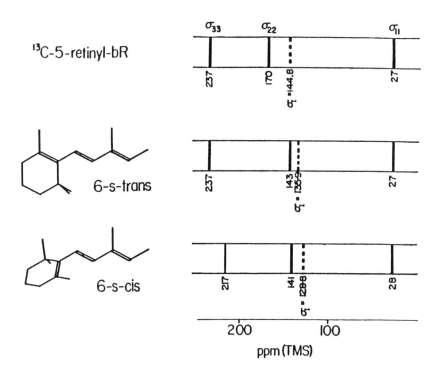

FIG. 3. Isotropic chemical shifts and shift tensor elements for the ^{13}C–5 positions of 6–s–<u>cis</u> and 6–s–<u>trans</u> retinoic acids together with similar data for ^{13}C–5–retinal–bR. In going from 6–s–<u>cis</u> to 6–s–<u>trans</u> only the σ_{33} element changes. The σ_{11} and and σ_{33} elements in bR indicate that the retinal in the protein is 6–s–<u>trans</u>. The movement in σ_{22} is attributed to the point charge.

which we can obtain the anisotropy are also indicated. The results of the Herzfeld–Berger analysis of these data are shown in Figure 3 for ^{13}C–5–bR together with two model compounds, 6–s–<u>trans</u> and 6–s–<u>cis</u> retinoic acid. We have performed similar experiments for 13 other retinal positions and the isotropic chemical shifts are summarized in Table I. We will discuss the interpretation of these results in the next section.

Figure 4 shows an ^{15}N MASS NMR spectrum obtained from hydrated bR containing ϵ–^{15}N–Lys. The line on the right (fwhm = 17 Hz) is due to the six free lysines of the protein and with resolution enhancement is split into a quartet. The strong band downfield from the lysine resonance is due to the natural–abundance amide backbone and the small doublet on the left arises from the Schiff base nitrogen, the splitting being due to the presence

TABLE I.   Chemical shifts of the 13–cis and all–trans isomers of bR, compared with those of all–trans–retinylidene butylimmonium chloride, in the solid state and solution

	bR_{568}	bR_{548}	NRBH+Cl−Solid[6]	NRBH+Cl−Solution[19]
C–5	144.8	144.8[5]	128.7	131.8
C–6	135.4	134.9[5]a	138.8	137.4
C–7	129.5	130.7[5]	128.8	132.0
C–8	132.7	131.6[5]	140.8	136.9
C–9	146.4	148.4[5]	142.1	145.3
C–10	133.0	129.7[4]	135.0	129.5
C–11	139.1	135.4[4]	138.9	137.4
C–12	134.3	124.2[4]	135.0	133.6
C–13	169.0	165.3[5]a	161.8	162.3
C–14	122.0	110.5[3]	122.5	120.1
C–15	163.2	160.4[5]a	167.0	163.6
C–18	22.0	22.0[5]	23.3	21.9
C–19	11.3	11.3[4]	14.0	13.2
C–20	13.3	13.3[4]	14.0	14.3

* Numbers in parentheses are reference numbers.

a assignment to bR_{548} or bR_{568} is not known.

of all–trans and 13–cis retinal isomers in dark–adapted bR. The chemical shifts of these two components are listed in Table II together with data from some model compounds.

DISCUSSION

1. Configuration of the $C_{13}=C_{14}$ Bond

It is known from chemical extraction experiments that dark–adapted bR contains a mixture of all–trans and 13–cis retinal PSB isomers in an approximate 4:6 ratio (17).   These two configurations can easily be detected in the NMR spectra by the presence of two lines in all of the ^{13}C spectra of retinals with labels in the polyene chain (3–6).   The results are

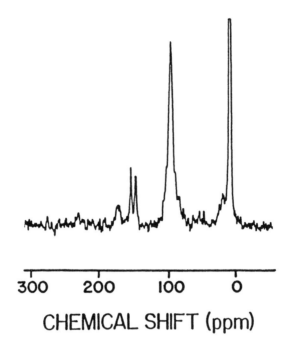

CHEMICAL SHIFT (ppm)

FIG. 4. ^{15}N MASS NMR spectrum of fully hydrated bR. The three lines are (from left to right) due to the Schiff base, the natural–abundance amide backbone, and the six additional lysines in the protein. The Schiff base doublet arises from the presence of 13–<u>cis</u>- and all–<u>trans</u>-retinal and the chemical shift indicates a protonated linkage which is weakly hydrogen–bonded.

quite similar to the ^{15}N spectra shown in Figure 5. The fact that the 13–<u>cis</u> isomer is present in bR is confirmed by examining the chemical shift of the 12–carbon which is moved upfield by ~10 ppm on isomerization (1,18). This upfield shift is due to a γ–effect and the shift has been observed to be totally resident in the σ_{11} element of the shift tensor in two polyene systems (6,13,22). In bR we also observed an upfield shift for C–12 (124.2 ppm) as shown in Table I. As in the case with the model compounds, this shift is largely resident in the σ_{11} shift tensor element, confirming that it is due to a γ–effect on all–<u>trans</u> to 13–<u>cis</u> isomerization. The presence of all–<u>trans</u> and 13–<u>cis</u> retinals is illustrated in Figure 5.

2. Configuration of the C=N Bond

We also observe an upfield shift of 12 ppm for one of the C–14 lines as shown in Table I. Moreover, measurement of the sideband intensities shows that this shift is primarily due to changes in the σ_{11} element and therefore a γ–effect is probably also responsible for this shift (3). In order for a γ–effect to occur, there must be a steric interaction between the proton

Table II.   Isotropic Shifts Derived from MASS (σ_I) and Static Powder Spectra [1/3 Tr (σ)] along with Chemical Shift Tensor Elements Obtained from Powder Spectra[a] (2)

Sample	σ_I	1/3 Tr ($\tilde{\sigma}$)	σ_{11}	σ_{22}	σ_{33}
^{15}N–RB	315.3	314.9	11.5	309.6	623.6
^{15}N–RBH$^+$Cl$^-$	171.7	172.5	27.3	194.6	296.3
^{15}N–RBH$^+$Br$^-$	166.1	165.5	26.7	183.3	286.6
^{15}N–RB$^+$I$^-$	154.4	154.6	26.3	163.8	273.8
^{15}N–Lys–bR					
Schiff base	144.9 151.6	(av 148.3)			
Amide backbone	93.6				
ε–Lys–^{15}NH$_3^+$	8.4				

[a] Estimated errors are ±1 ppm for the tensor elements and ±0.2 ppm for MASS isotropic shifts. All shifts are downfield from external 5.6 M ^{15}NH$_4$Cl in H$_2$O.

attached to C–14 and protons on a carbon three bonds away. As shown in Figure 5 a likely candidate is the ε–carbon of the Lys sidechain, provided the C=N bond is in a syn (or cis) configuration. We assign the C=N syn bond to the 13–cis component of the dark–adapted spectrum based on the relative intensities of the two observed spectral lines. As noted above, chemical extraction experiments indicate the 13–cis/all–trans ratio is ~6:4 and the spectral line intensities follow this pattern.

The reason(s) for formation of the 13–cis, 15–syn conformation will remain unclear until more is known about the structure of the chromophore in the other photocycle intermediates. However, it would appear that a potential motivation for this conformational change is that it provides a mechanism for 13–cis formation that does not require large excursions of the β–ionone ring portion of the retinal. The presence of a single cis bond at the 13–position creates a situation in which the retinal from carbon–13 to the carbon–5 would have to swing through ~60° when the C$_{13}$=C$_{14}$ bond isomerizes to the cis configuration. However, with the 15–syn formation this portion of the molecule simply moves laterally as is illustrated in Figure 5. 13–cis, 15–syn formation in retinal Schiff bases is analogous to formation of a gtg' "kink" in a polymethylene chain. A single gauche bond would lead to a large 60° displacement of the remaining part of the chain. However, formation of the kink reduces this movement to a small lateral displacement of the chain.

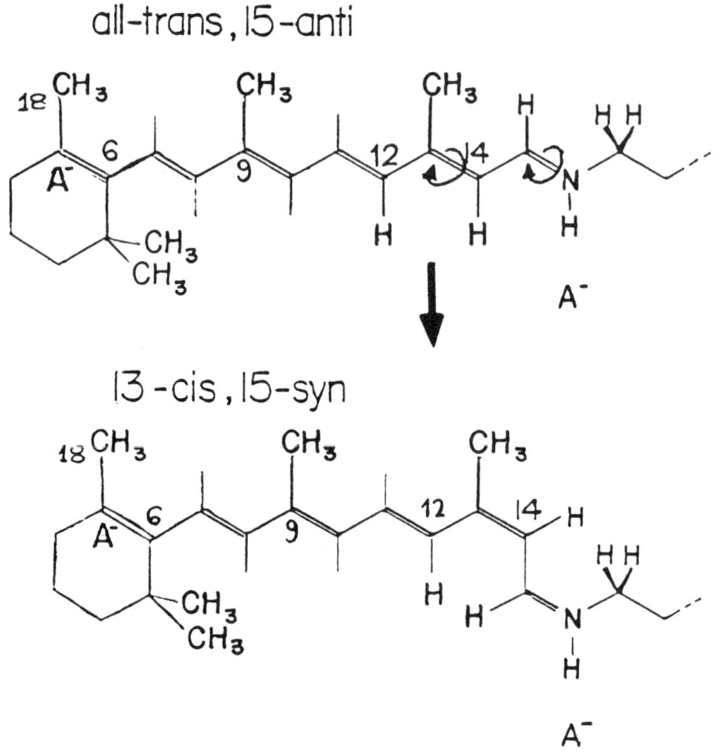

FIG. 5. Retinal Schiff base illustrating the features of its conformation in dark–adapted bR determined from the ^{13}C and ^{15}N MASS NMR spectra. They are: (a) cis and trans conformations at the 13 bond; (b) syn and anti C=N bonds; (c) 6–s–trans bonds and a perturbing point charge in both 13–cis and all–trans forms, and (d) a protonated Schiff base linkage which is weakly hydrogen–bonded.

3. Conformation about the 6–s–Bond and the Opsin Shift

It is generally assumed that the most stable conformation of the retinal chromophore in solution, in bR, and in rhodopsin is the 6–s–cis form (9). Protonated retinal Schiff bases formed from the 6–s–cis retinal conformers have an absorption maximum around 440 nm which is shifted to ~570 nm in bR and to ~500 nm in rhodopsin by a protein perturbation –– the "opsin shift". It was initially suggested that the protein perturbation responsible for the shift in rhodopsin is an electrostatic charge (11) and recent evidence has supported this idea for bacteriorhodopsin (14,15). The ^{13}C MASS NMR experiments permit us to test and refine this concept further.

As shown in Figure 3 the chemical shift of ^{13}C–5 permits us to distinguish between the 6–s–cis and 6–s–trans forms of retinal. By studying two forms of retinoic acid which crystallize in the 6–s–cis and 6–s–trans forms, we were able to show that the C–5 isotropic shift moves downfield by 7 ppm (129 ppm → 136 ppm) on going from cis to trans (6). Furthermore, an analysis of the shift anisotropies from the sideband patterns shows that the effect is localized in the downfield σ_{33} element — it moves 20 ppm — (recall the γ–effect results primarily in a shift of the upfield σ_{11} element). σ_{11} and σ_{22} are essentially unchanged by this isomerization, as shown in Figure 3.

In bR the isotropic and anisotropic shifts are both similar and different. As shown in Figure 3, σ_{11} = 27 ppm and σ_{33} = 237 ppm in both 6–s–trans retinoic acid and in bR. These data, together with the T_1 of the ^{13}C–18 (methyl group) and the isotropic shift at C–8, indicate that bR contains a 6–s–trans retinal chromophore (5). However, we observe an additional 27 ppm downfield movement in σ_{22} which we believe is due to the presence of a point charge in the neighborhood of the β–ionone ring. Although other positions in the β–ionone ring of retinal remain to be studied (C–1 through C–4), the observation of a large shift in σ_{22} at C–5 provides strong experimental evidence for the location of the putative point charge. This location agrees quite well with the work of Honig and Nakanishi based on optical spectra (14). Note that both the 13–cis and all–trans retinals are shown in a 6–s–trans form in Figure 5 and the point charge is located adjacent to C–5.

Finally, we should mention that the occurrence of a 6–s–trans conformer in bR has another important ramification for our understanding of the opsin shift. In particular, it has been assumed that the 5100 cm^{-1} shift is due to a point charge near the β–ionone ring of a 6–s–cis conformer. However, Honig et al. (10) have calculated that a 6–s–cis to 6–s–trans conformational change can account for about one–third of this shift. Thus, the NMR data suggest that a significant fraction of the opsin shift is not due to the point charge.

4. Protonation State of the Schiff Base

The ^{15}N chemical shift of Schiff bases is extraordinarily sensitive to their state of protonation. As we have shown elsewhere (2), there is an ~150 ppm shift (from 300 to 150 ppm) of the isotropic line on protonation of a retinal N–butylamine Schiff base. Concurrently, the shift anisotropy spectrum changes from an η ≈ 1 powder pattern with a breadth of 600 ppm to an η ≈ 0.5 pattern with a breadth of 270 ppm. Thus, a simple measurement of the isotropic or anisotropic shifts is sufficient to distinguish between a protonated and an unprotonated Schiff base. The average chemical shift shown in Figure 4 is 148 ppm and is clearly much closer to protonated (σ_I ~154–172) rather than unprotonated (σ_I ~315 ppm) Schiff bases.

In addition, there are two other interesting features in the spectrum of Figure 4. First, as mentioned above, is the doublet splitting of 7 ppm which is due to the presence of the 13–cis and all–trans isomers present in dark–adapted bR. A similar splitting is also observed in ^{13}C spectra at essentially all other positions along the polyene chain — only at position 5 of the β–ionone ring is the splitting not observable. Second, the chemical shifts of the bR Schiff base lines are 145 and 152 ppm, which are further upfield than even the iodide salt of N–butyl retinal (Table II). We have performed a thorough investigation of the dependence of ^{15}N Schiff base chemical shifts on hydrogen bonding strength (7). Specifically, using two–dimensional dipolar/ chemical shift experiments we have measured bond distances in a number of protonated Schiff bases where the ^{15}N chemical shifts span a range of 150–170 ppm. The data show a clear linear correlation between ^{15}N chemical shift, shift anisotropies, and the NH bond distance. The weaker the hydrogen bond, the farther upfield the chemical shift. Thus, the ^{15}N spectra show the Schiff base to be protonated, to be weakly hydrogen–bonded, and they show the coexistence of 13–cis and all–trans retinals. The protonated Schiff base linkage in both the all–trans and 13–cis forms of retinal together with the weak hydrogen bond are illustrated in Figure 5.

CONCLUSIONS

The experiments discussed here constitute one of the first thorough MASS NMR studies of a protein, and as such, illustrate some of the types of results which can be gleaned from such an effort. For example, it has been possible to characterize in some detail the conformation of the active site of a protein by incorporating ^{13}C and ^{15}N labels into the system. With this ability a number of new features of retinal structures have emerged as well as better understanding of the opsin shift. The experiments also illustrate the utility of examining sidebands and shift anisotropies rather than confining one's attention to the "traditional" isotropic chemical shifts. In particular, the changes in shift tensor elements provide a much clearer picture of the conformation and electrostatic environment of retinal than do the isotropic shifts alone. We anticipate that this type of investigation should now be feasible for a number of other membrane and crystalline proteins.

ACKNOWLEDGMENTS

The authors gratefully acknowledge the assistance in retinal synthesis of Gerard't Lam (^{13}C–6 and ^{13}C–7), Ellen van den Berg (^{13}C–8 and ^{13}C–9) and Toon Peters (^{13}C–18). This research was supported by the U.S. National Institutes of Health (GM–23316, GM–23289, EY–02051, and RR–00995), the U.S. National Science Foundation (CHE–8116042 and DMR–8211416), the Netherlands Foundation for Chemical Research (SON) and the Netherlands Organization for the Advancement of Pure Research (ZWO). R.A.M. is a recipient of an NIH Research Career Development Award.

REFERENCES

1. Becker, R.S., Berger, S., Dalling, D.K., Grant, D.M., and Pugmire, R. (1974): J. Am. Chem. Soc. 96:7008–7014.
2. Harbison, G.S., Herzfeld, J. and Griffin, R.G. (1983): Biochemistry 22:1–5.
3. Harbison, G.S. Smith, S.O., Pardoen, J.A., Winkel, C., Lugtenburg, J., Herzfeld, J., Mathies, R. and Griffin, R.G. (1984): Proc. Natl. Acad. Sci. USA 81:1706–1709.
4. Harbison, G.S., Smith, S.O., Pardoen, J.A., Mulder, P.P.J., Lugtenburg, J., Herzfeld, J., Mathies, R. and Griffin, R.G. (1984): Biochemistry 23:2662–2667.
5. Harbison, G., Smith, S.O., Pardoen, J.A., Courtin, J.M.L., Lugtenburg, J., Herzfeld, J., Mathies, R.A. and Griffin, R.G. (1985): Biochemistry 24:6955–6962.
6. Harbison, G.S., Mulder, P.P.J., Pardoen, J.A., Lugtenburg, J., Herzfeld, J. and Griffin, R.G. (1985): J. Am. Chem. Soc. 107:4809–4816.
7. Harbison, G.S., Roberts, J.E., Herzfeld, J. and Griffin, R.G. (1985): Biochemistry, to be submitted.
8. Herzfeld, J. and Berger, A.E. (1980): J. Chem. Phys. 73:6021–6030.
9. Honig, B., Hudson, B., Sykes, B.D. and Karplus, M. (1971): Proc. Natl. Acad. Sci. USA 68:1289–1293.
10. Honig, B., Greenberg, A., Dinur, U. and Ebrey, T.G. (1976):Biochemistry 15:4593–4599.
11. Kropf, A. and Hubbard, R. (1958): Ann. N.Y. Acad. Sci. 74:266–280.
12. Mateescu, G.D., Copan, W.G., Muccio, D.D., Waterhous, D.V. and Abrahamson, E.W. (1983): in "Proceedings of the International Symposium on Synthesis and Applications of Isotopically Labeled Compounds", pp. 123–132, Elsevier, Amsterdam.
13. Mehring, M., Weber, H., Muller, W. and Wegner, G. (1983): Solid State Comm. 45:1079–1082.
14. Nakanishi, K., Balogh–Nair, V., Arnaboldi, M., Tsujimoto, K. and Honig, B. (1980): J. Am. Chem. Soc. 102:7945–7947.
15. Nakanishi, K. (1985): Pure and Appl. Chem. 57:769–772.
16. Ottolenghi, M. (1980): Adv. Photochem. 12:97–200.
17. Pettei, M.J., Yudd, A.P., Nakanishi, K., Henselman, R. and Stoeckenius, W. (1977): Biochemistry 16:1955–1959.
18. Rowan, R. and Sykes, B.D. (1974): J. Am. Chem. Soc. 96:7000–7008.
19. Shriver, J. Abrahamson, E.W. and Mateescu, G.D. (1976): J. Am. Chem. Soc. 98:2407–2409.
20. Smith, S.O., Lugtenburg, J. and Mathies, R. (1985): J. Memb. Biol.85:95–109.
21. Stoeckenius, W. and Bogomolni, R.A. (1982): Ann. Rev. Biochem. 51:587–616.
22. Terao, T. Maeda, S., Yamabe, T., Akagi, K. and Shirakawa, H. (1984): Chem. Phys. Letters 102:347–352.
23. Yamaguchi, A., Unemoto, T. and Ikegami, A. (1981): Photochem. Photobiol. 33:511–516.

II. HIGH–RESOLUTION NMR OF BIOLOGICAL MACROMOLECULES

NMR in Biology and Medicine,
edited by Shu Chien and Chien Ho.
Raven Press, New York © 1986.

New Techniques in the Study of Biomolecular Structure by High Field NMR

A. A. Bothner–By

Carnegie–Mellon University, Pittsburgh, Pennsylvania 15213

The pace of technological advance in the application of high–resolution NMR to the investigation of biomolecular structure shows no signs of abating; rather it is accelerating with new, more powerful, more sensitive and more revealing techniques being invented and demonstrated daily. This is ascribable, in part, to the rapid progress being made in instrumentation and computer technology, in part to increasingly clear and comprehensible models and treatments of the phenomena involved, which allow the scientist to contrive sophisticated new experiments to meet new requirements with relative ease.

At the NMR Facility for Biomedical Studies in Pittsburgh, we have been interested particularly in the application of high resolution NMR using the highest attainable field, and for the past five years, have been working with a spectrometer incorporating a super–conducting solenoid generating a field of 14.09 T, corresponding to a frequency of 600 MHz for protons, 243 MHz for ^{31}P, etc. Many spectra have been obtained confirming the expected usefulness of the high field as a result of its greater spectral dispersion and sensitivity. The advance to higher field also brings new problems and opportunities with it. In meeting these, we have contributed to the development of new techniques, either to ameliorate the problems, or to exploit the opportunities. In this talk, we will discuss two examples: first a problem, second an opportunity.

OVERHAUSER EFFECTS

Longitudinal and Transverse

The value of the nuclear Overhauser effect for structural investigations became widely appreciated following the appearance of a monograph on the subject by Noggle and Schirmer (17). The effect is defined as the change in integrated intensity of the NMR signal from one set of nuclei, resulting from nonequilibrium magnetization of a second set. It occurs as a result of cross–relaxation between nuclei of the two sets. If we symbolize the longitudinal magnetizations of the homonuclear sets A and B by m_A and m_B and their equilibrium magnetizations by m_0, we can write

$$\dot{m}_A = -\rho_1(m_A - m_0) - \sigma_1(m_B - m_0) \qquad [1]$$

$$\dot{m}_B = -\sigma_1(m_A - m_0) - \rho_1(m_B - m_0) \qquad [2]$$

Here ρ_1 and σ_1 are the auto–relaxation and cross–relaxation rate constants. These differential equations may be solved quite easily for various types of experiments. For example, if the resonance of B is saturated in a homonuclear AB system, $m_B = 0$, and setting $\dot{m}_A = 0$ in equation [1] in order to obtain the steady state solution, we get

$$0 = -\rho_1(m_A - m_0) + \sigma_1 m_0 \qquad [3]$$

or

$$m_A = [1 + (\sigma_1/\rho_1)]\, m_0 \qquad [4]$$

so that σ_1/ρ_1 represents the fractional change in intensity. From an analysis of longitudinal relaxation by direct nuclear magnetic dipole interaction, Solomon (19) evaluated σ_1 and ρ_1 as

$$\sigma_1 = K \left[\frac{6\tau_C}{1 + 4\omega^2\tau_C^2} - \tau_C \right] \qquad [5]$$

$$\rho_1 = K \left[\frac{6\tau_C}{1 + 4\omega^2\tau_C} + \frac{3\tau_C}{1 + \omega^2\tau_C^2} + \tau_C \right] \qquad [6]$$

Here K is a constant, $(\gamma^4 h^2/10 r^6_{AB})$, τ_C is the correlation time for reorientation of the A–B internuclear axis and ω is the nuclear Larmor frequency in radians/sec. Dividing equation [5] by equation [6] we get

$$\frac{\sigma_1}{\rho_1} = \frac{5 + \omega^2\tau_C^2 - 4\omega^4\tau_C^4}{10 + 23\omega^2\tau_C^2 + 4\omega^4\tau_C^4} \qquad [7]$$

We see immediately that if $\omega\tau_C \ll 1$ (i.e. if the molecules in solution tumble rapidly compared to the spectrometer frequency), the change in intensity in our experiment will be $+ 0.5\, m_0$, an increase of 50%. On the other hand, if $\omega^2\tau_C^2 \gg 1$ (high molecular weight molecules tumbling slowly, or high spectrometer frequency), the effect will be -1.0, corresponding to disappearance of the A signal. At some intermediate point, where $\omega^2\tau_C^2 = 5/4$, no effect will be detected. These considerations are now well understood and tested (3). The negative effects observed in high molecular weight compounds have been mapped using elegant two–dimensional methods in proteins (10) and nucleic acids (4), and have proven of great value in structural studies and spectral assignment. Some problems accompany the application of this method at high field, however.

Firstly, a variety of interesting biomolecules of intermediate molecular weight, such as peptides, antibiotics, and polysaccharides, have molecular weights in a range such that $\omega^2\tau_c^2 \simeq 5/4$ at 500 or 600 MHz, so that the longitudinal Overhauser effect is small and cannot be detected. Secondly, for high ω or τ_c such that $\omega\tau_c \gg 1$, the value of $\sigma/\rho = -1.0$ implies efficient transfer of magnetization from one nucleus to the next neighboring nucleus, such that in a large network of nuclei, the effect will be spread quickly throughout the network, and the specificity of the effects will be lost (9). In order to overcome this difficulty, observation of truncated or transient effects is performed. Only very short cross–relaxation times are used, preventing multi–spin effects. This decreases sensitivity, since small, short–time effects must be detected.

A technique for overcoming these problems consists in observing the cross–relaxation between the spins not in the longitudinal direction, as has been customary, but in the transverse direction. Equations [1] and [2] must be modified to

$$\dot{m}_A = -\rho_2 m_A - \sigma_2 m_B \qquad\qquad [8]$$

$$\dot{m}_B = -\sigma_2 m_A - \rho_2 m_B \qquad\qquad [9]$$

with m_A and m_B now representing the <u>transverse</u> magnetizations, and

$$\rho_2 = K\,[2.5\tau_c + \frac{4.5\tau_c}{1 + \omega\tau_c} + \frac{3\tau_c}{1 + 4\omega\tau_c}] \qquad\qquad [10]$$

$$\sigma_2 = K\,[2\tau_c + \frac{3\tau_c}{1 + \omega^2\tau_c^2}] \qquad\qquad [11]$$

which gives

$$\frac{\sigma_2}{\rho_2} = \frac{10 + 44\omega^2\tau_c^2 + 16\omega^4\tau_c^4}{20 + 67\omega^2\tau_c^2 + 20\omega^4\tau_c^4} \qquad\qquad [12]$$

This gives $\sigma_2/\rho_2 = +0.5$, as before, if $\omega_2\tau_c^2 \ll 1$, but $\sigma_2/\rho_2 = +0.8$, if $\omega_2\tau_c^2 \gg 1$. The effect lies between these limits for all values of $\omega_2\tau_c^2$, so the difficulties of near zero effects for intermediate molecular weights and spin diffusion for high molecular weights does not occur.

As an example of the application of this technique, let us consider the solution conformations of two substances related to erythromycin. This macrolide antibiotic, produced by <u>streptomyces</u> <u>erythreus</u> is medicinally important (15), has been studied by a wide variety of methods (16), and has been recently synthesized (21). A very interesting observation, made during the synthetic effort, was that the closure of the 14–membered lactone ring (Formula 1) proceeded in excellent yield with the precursor seco–9S–dihydroerythronolide A bis(3,5)(9,11) mesityl acetal, (the open form), but in small or zero yield with a number of derivatives with differently disposed protecting groups. A possible explanation is that the acetal formation in this case constrains the open form in a conformation which is close to that of the closed form, so that cyclization can readily take place. It seemed to us of interest to explore this question by attempting to obtain evidence for the conformations of the open and closed forms in solution.

The 600 MHz spectrum of the closed form is shown in Figure 1 with peak assignments obtained in a straightforward way by spin–decoupling experiments. The chemical shifts and coupling constants found for both open and closed forms are given in Table 1.

Specific effects between protons were first sought by individual 1–D experiments. The protocol for performing these experiments was:

1. Obtain a reference spectrum without Overhauser effects by applying a $90°_x$ nonselective pulse, followed with no delay by application of a spin–locking r.f. field along y with 0.25 seconds duration, and subsequent collection of the f.i.d.

2. Obtain a perturbed spectrum, by preliminary selective inversion of a particular signal, using a soft pulse, then proceeding as in 1.

3. Form a difference spectrum between the results of 1 and 2.

Since the equilibrium transverse magnetization is zero, one cannot perform a steady state experiment as commonly performed for the longitudinal Overhauser effect. However, the spin locking time may be chosen to give the maximum observable effect, and this is equal to about 3/4 of σ_2/ρ_2. Figure 1 displays difference spectra obtained in this way with selective inversion of the proton on C3, C5 and C11. The difference spectra show clear cross ring effects for example H5–H8 and H11–H4.

Formula 1: View of conformation suggested for erythronolide A bis mesityl acetal, closed form.

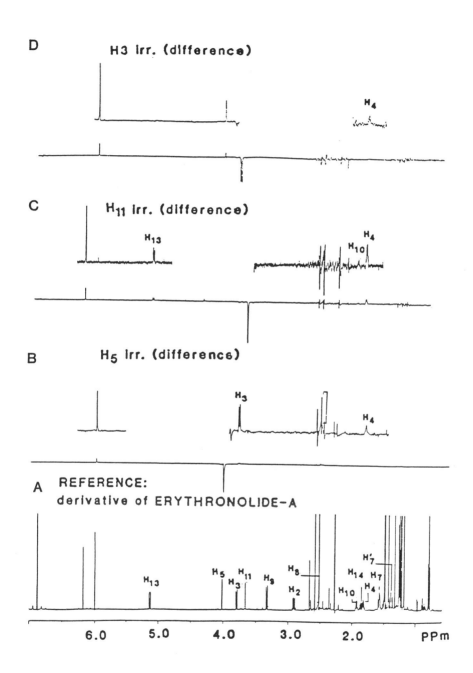

FIG. 1. CAMELSPIN reference (A) and difference (B,C,D) spectra of the closed form of erythronolide A bis mesityl acetal. 250 msec spin locking time.

Table 1. Spectral Assignments, Erythronolide A
Bis Mesityl Acetal

Nuclei	Closed Form		Open Form	
	Chemical Shift* (ppm)	Coupling Constant (Hz)	Chemical Shift* (ppm)	Coupling Constant (Hz)
H2	2.94	$J_{2,3}$; 11.5	2.85	$J_{2,3}$; 10.6
H3	3.82	$J_{3,4}$; 1.98	3.88	$J_{3,4}$; 2.3
H4	1.86	$J_{4,5}$; 2.36	1.85	$J_{4,5}$; 2.3
H5	4.04	---	3.60	---
H7	1.62	$J_{7,7'}$; 14.7	1.52	$J_{7,7'}$; 15.0
H7'	1.40	$J_{7',8}$; 11.5	1.25	$J_{7',8}$; 6.40
H8	2.50	$J_{8,9}$; 11.5	2.56	$J_{8,9}$; 11.4
H9	3.36	$J_{9,10}$; <1.0	3.28	$J_{9,10}$; <1.0
H10	1.96	$J_{10,11}$; 2.64	1.95	$J_{10,11}$; 2.30
H11	3.69	---	4.25	---
H13	5.15	$J_{13,14}$; 11.3	3.20	$J_{13,14}$; 10.5
H14	1.86	$J_{13,14'}$; 2.37	1.70	$J_{14,14}$; 13.7
H14'	1.51	---	1.25	---

* Reference: $CHCl_3$ at 7.28 ppm.

The reference spectrum and difference spectra with inversion of protons on the C-12 CH_3, C4, and the 9,11 acetal carbon are shown in Figure 2 for the open form.

In the study of this and of more complicated cases, a 2-D method offers advantages in economy of observation time and in compact data presentation. The expansion of the technique to a 2-D version is practical and offers some interesting points. The protocol for a basic 2-D experiment (called a CAMELSPIN experiment) is:

    1. Application of a $90°_x$ pulse, turning all nuclei to the $-y$ direction.

    2. Evolution for a time t_1, during which the spins dephase according to their chemical shifts and couplings.

    3. Application of the locking field for a time τ_m, the cross–relaxation time. The field clamps the components parallel to it, while those perpendicular are rapidly destroyed because of the inhomogeneity of H.

    4. Removal of the locking field and acquisition of the f.i.d. during t_2.

    Two dimensional Fourier transformation with respect to t_2 and t_1 provides a 2D–spectrum with the unperturbed spectrum along the diagonal, and cross–peaks corresponding to transverse nuclear Overhauser effects. Figure 3 shows such a spectrum for the closed form. Numerous effects are visible. Effects observed in both 1–D and 2–D experiments are listed in Table 2 for the open and closed forms.

    The description and theory given above are accurate for uncoupled systems. The presence of strong spin–spin splitting introduces complications in both the longitudinal and transverse Overhauser effect experiments which must be treated separately. In either 2–D NOESY or the CAMELSPIN experiment, it often happens that at the end of the evolution period spin multiplets will have evolved so that the components are no longer in phase. Application of the mixing and observe pulses in NOESY or the spin locking field in CAMELSPIN produces, in this case, coherent transfer of magnetization from one set of coupled spins to the other, and this is revealed in the form of J cross–peaks in the spectrum. Several ways of partially suppressing these have been suggested (13). A method, which is completely effective for AX systems, has been developed for CAMELSPIN.

    We illustrate this for the particularly simple system of cinnamic acid. Figure 4A shows the basic 2–D CAMELSPIN spectrum, which illustrates the occurrence of large cross–peaks, labeled J between the trans–olefinic protons, coupled with a 15.2 Hz spin–spin interaction. Spectrum 4B was taken with a modified sequence, in which the original $90°_x$–t_1 – excitation has been replaced with a $90°_x$–$t_{1/2}$–$180°_x$–$t_{1/2}$–$90°_y$–t_1– excitation. The $90°_y$ pulse has the effect of reversing the labels on the spin multiplets (20), so that they are exactly refocused at the end of the evolution period, t_1. The chemical shifts, which had been refocused by the $180°_x$ pulse at the time of the $90°_y$ pulse, evolve during t_1 in the normal way. The action of the spin locking field on the system with multiplet components in–phase produces no mixing, so no J cross–peak is observed.

    Consideration of the effects listed in Table 2 for the closed and open forms of the erythronolide A derivatives, in particular the cross–ring effects, as well as of the proton–proton coupling constants in each, allow the postulation of reasonable conformations for each. In the proposed conformation of the closed form there are two transoid chains, composed of C2–C3–C4–C5–C6 and C9–C10–C11–C12–C13, joined by loops consisting of C6–C7–C8 and the lactone portion. A rendering of the suggested conformation is given in Formula 1. From the similarity of all coupling constants (except between protons on C7 and C8) the open form appears to have a similar conformation, but the opening of the lactone linkage allows the two branches to move slightly apart, by rotation about bonds C7–C8 and possibly C6–C7 reducing the cross–ring CAMELSPIN

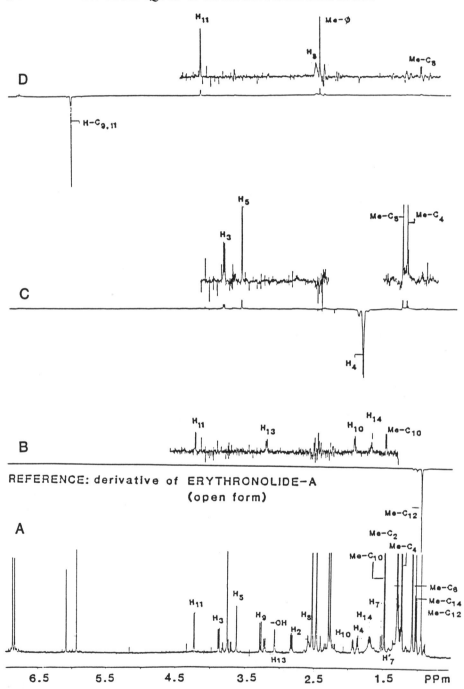

FIG. 2. CAMELSPIN reference (A) and difference (B,C,D) spectra of the open form of erythronolide A bis mesityl acetal. 250 msecs. spin locking time.

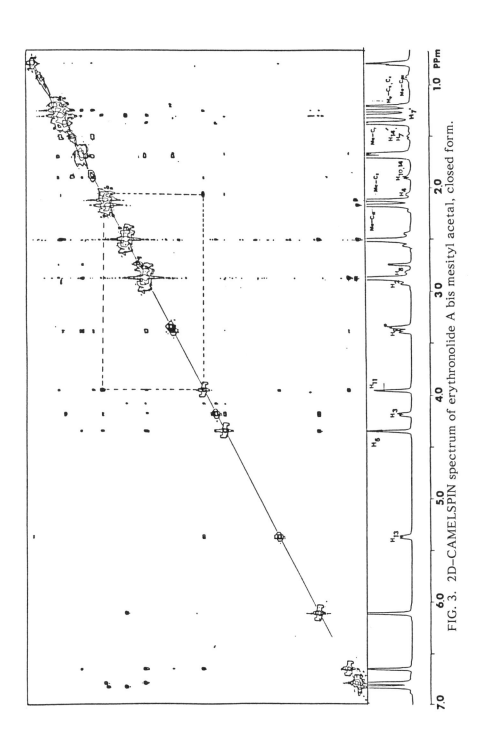

FIG. 3. 2D–CAMELSPIN spectrum of erythronolide A bis mesityl acetal, closed form.

effects. In addition, the terminal chain C12–C13–C14 adopts a different population of rotamers in the open form. Thus, only a small reorganization is required for cyclization.

Table 2.   Comparison of Transverse Nuclear Overhauser Effects between the Open Form and the Closed Form of Erythronolide A Bis Mesityl Acetal

Irradiated Nuclei	Open Form NOE at	Closed Form NOE at
H(9,11)*	H11, 35.0 H8, 16.5 Me–aromatic, 1.0 Me–C8 —	H11, 27.0 H8, — Me–aromatic 1.0
H(3,5)*	H3, 16.8 H5, 14.7 Me–aromatic 2.0	H3, 23.0 H5, 19.0 Me–aromatic 1.5
H3	H3,5 25.0 H5, 3.0 H4, 8.0 Me–C2 1.0	H3,5 32.0 H5, 10.0 H4, 6.0 Me–C2 small
H4	H3, 8.0 H5, 12.0 Me–C4, small Me–C6 small	----
H5	H3,5 25.0 H4, 8.0 H3, small H7 5.0	H3,5 35.0 H3, 11.0 H8, 1.1 H4 8.0
H9	H10, 6.0 H7, 13.0 Me–C10, 1.0 Me–C8 2.0	H10, 4.0 Me–C10, 2.0 H7' 3.0
H10	H11, 11.0 H9, 6.0 Me–C10, 1.0 Me–C12 small	H11, 2.0 H9, 3.0 Me–C10, 3.0 Me–C12 small
H11	H9,11 40.0 H8, 9.0 H10, 10.0 Me–C10, 2.5 H14 2.5	H9,11 40.0 H13, 8.0 H4, 30.0 H10, 5.5 H8 small
Me–C12	H11, 9.0 H13, 6.7 H10, 22.0 H14, — Me–C10 —	----

* Acetyl protons

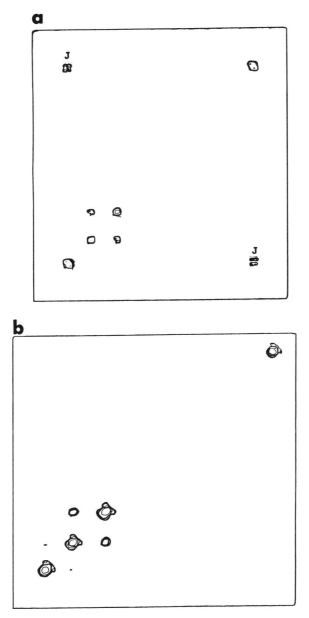

Fig. 4. 2D–CAMELSPIN of cinnamic acid with basic (a) and modified (b) excitation schemes. The J cross–peak labeled J in a, is eliminated in b.

MOLECULAR ALIGNMENT

Strong Fields and Anisotropic Molecules

The interpretation of high resolution NMR spectra of molecules in the liquid state has been based on the assumption that the molecules tumble completely randomly in solution. The high resolution Hamiltonian, with this assumption, leads to the well known rules (18) that spin–spin splitting is independent of static field strength, that coupling between magnetically equivalent spin –1/2 nuclei cannot be observed, that chemical shifts are proportional to the applied static field, and that quadrupole coupling does not yield an observable splitting in the signals of quadrupolar nuclei.

When molecules are oriented, as in solids or liquid crystalline solution, or by the action of some other agency, these rules no longer apply (6). Direct magnetic dipolar interaction between the nuclei contributes to the splitting, and, as the degree of orientation varies, the observed splitting varies. Splitting between magnetically equivalent nuclei can be observed. Quadrupole splitting is observed in the signals of quadrupolar nuclei.

Recently in our laboratories and in those of Prof. C. MacLean, Amsterdam, it has been shown that fields of 10 Tesla or more orient certain molecules sufficiently that direct dipolar interactions (8) and quadrupole splittings (11) can be detected and measured in the normal high resolution spectrum. This provides an interesting new tool for the investigation of molecular geometry, aggregation, and electronic properties in solution.

The partial alignment of the molecules occurs as a result of the interaction of the strong static magnetic field with the anisotropic magnetic susceptibility of the individual molecules. If a molecule has an anisotropic susceptibility tensor χ, with principal axes x,y,z, the energy of the molecule immersed in a field, H_0, is given by

$$E = -1/2 \quad H_0 \cdot \underset{\sim}{\chi} \cdot H_0 \qquad [13]$$

so that the energy will depend on the orientation of the molecule in the field. In this lecture we will concentrate on molecules with exact or approximate axial symmetry, so that $\chi_{xx} = \chi_{yy} \neq \chi_{zz}$, and we will define $\Delta\chi = \chi_{zz} - \chi_{xx} = \chi_{zz} - \chi_{yy}$. If we suppose that the molecular energies given in [13] follow a Boltzmann distribution, we obtain

$$S_{zz} = H^2 \, \Delta\chi/15kT \qquad [14]$$

Here $S_{zz} = 1/2 \, <3\cos^2\theta_{zz} - 1>$, is the orientation parameter defined by Saupe (14), and θ_{zz} is the angle between the z axis of the molecular susceptibility tensor and the static magnetic field.

We are interested in S_{kl}, the degree of alignment of a particular internuclear axis (k,l) in the molecule. This axis may or may not be coincident with the z axis of the molecular susceptibility tensor. In order to obtain S_{kl}, we use the relation

$$S_{kl} = S_{zz} (3 \cos^2\alpha - 1)/2 \qquad\qquad [15]$$

where α is the angle between the molecular z axis and the axis joining k and l.

If the nuclei k,l are both magnetic, a direct dipolar interaction, D_{kl} will be observed, given by

$$D_{kl} = - S_{kl} (\gamma_k\gamma_l\, h/2\pi^2 r_{kl}^3) \qquad\qquad [16]$$

For an AX case, the splitting observed (6) will be $J_{kl}+D_{kl}$, while for equivalent nuclei, the splitting will be $3D_{kl}/2$. Combining equations 14, 15 and 16, and simplifying, we get the practical equation:

$$D_{kl} = - 3.20 \times 10^{12}\, \nu_k\nu_l\, \Delta\chi(3\cos^2\alpha - 1)/a^3 T \qquad\qquad [17]$$

where ν_k and ν_l are the spectrometer frequencies in Hertz for k and l, and a is the internuclear distance in Ångstroms.

If k,l represent, for example, ^{12}C and ^2H nuclei, it may be assumed that the electric field gradient is axial and parallel to the bond, and a quadrupole splitting of the ^2H signal will be observed (22) given by

$$\delta\nu = \frac{3}{2} \left(\frac{e^2qQ}{h}\, S_{kl}\right) \qquad\qquad [18]$$

Anisotropic magnetic susceptibilities are a common feature of aromatic compounds, acetylenic compounds, halogenated compounds, etc. Some illustrations of the effect of orientation on the deuteron spectra of simple compounds are given in Figure 5.

Substituting in equation 18 the accepted value of 186 KHz for (e^2qQ/h) for aromatically–bound deuterons, and taking account of the D_{6h} symmetry of benzene, we obtain a value of $\Delta\chi$ for benzene of -1.02×10^{-28} cm^3/molecule. This is in excellent agreement with measurements made by Cotton–Mouton effects (2), solid state crystal measurements (12), and microwave Zeeman effect (7) measurements on related compounds. The observed splitting in C^2HCl_3 allows the calculation of $\Delta\chi$ for $^2HCCl_3$ as $+0.23 \times 10^{-28}$ cm^3/molecule, a value apparently not previously measured, and surprisingly large.

Numerous molecules of biological interest are expected to have significant molecular anisotropic susceptibilities, including nucleic acids, and porphyrins such as hemes and chlorophyll derivatives. To illustrate the application of this kind of study to such molecules, we will consider the case of vinylphylloerythrin methyl ester, Formula 2, a derivative of chlorophyll.

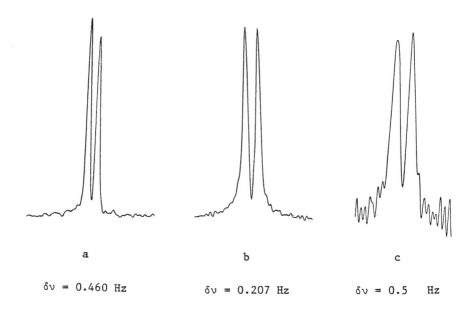

a

$\delta \nu = 0.460$ Hz

b

$\delta \nu = 0.207$ Hz

c

$\delta \nu = 0.5$ Hz

FIG. 5. Quadrupole splittings observed in the 92.2 MHz ^{2}H NMR spectrum of (a) benzene–^{2}H$_1$ (with proton decoupling), (b) ^{2}HCCl$_3$, (c) ^{2}HCI$_3$, both in cyclohexane solution.

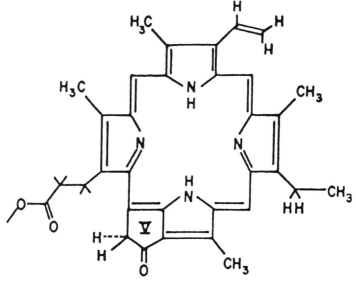

Formula 2. Vinylphylloerythrin methyl ester

It is first necessary to establish an acceptable value of $\Delta\chi$ for the porphyrin ring in the compound so that the degree of orientation may be determined. An indicator for this is the dipolar splitting, $(3/2)D_{kl}$, which appears in the signal from the CH_2 group of ring V. Porphyrins are known to aggregate strongly, and it is necessary to make the measurement under conditions where such aggregation is suppressed. For this purpose, Abraham, et al. (1) recommend observation of the Zn-complex in the presence of nitrogen-base, which coordinates with the Zn. The CH_2 doublet splitting observed under these conditions is shown in Figure 6, and amounts to 1.98 Hz at 600 MHz. Since the molecule has an average plane of symmetry bisecting the CH_2 group, the H-H internuclear axis is parallel to the z-axis. We take r_{HH} as 1.78 Å yielding, via equation 17, $\Delta\chi = - 9.5$ x 10^{-28} cm^3/molecule. Correcting for the coordinated pyridine molecule we get $\Delta\chi$ (porphyrin) = -10.0 x 10^{-28} cm^3/molecule.

If uncomplexed vinylphylloerythrin at 0.01M concentration in chloroform is examined, the splitting observed for the CH_2 group is 2.66 Hz at 600 MHz. The increase is ascribed to the formation of dimers which are more strongly aligned than the monomers. Dimer formation in porphyrins is by face-to-face association (5), so that the molecular z axes of the partners are parallel. Under these circumstances, $\Delta\chi$ for the dimer is just twice that for the monomer, and the dimeric pair will have S_{kl} values twice as large. If the fraction of porphyrin molecules dimerized is f_2, then the observed D_2 will be related to the splitting for the monomer D_1 by

$$D_2 = D_1(1 + f_2) \qquad\qquad [19]$$

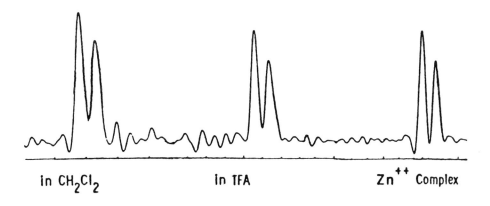

in CH_2Cl_2 In TFA Zn^{++} Complex

FIG. 6. Dipole-dipole splitting in the CH_2 signal of vinylphylloerythrin methyl ester in chloroform solution.

We conclude that the porphyrin in this solution is approximately 30% in the form of dimers.

The vinyl group in vinylphylloerythrin may rotate about the bond joining it to the porphyrin ring. We will characterize the rotation by the dihedral angle θ between the planes of the vinyl group and the porphyrin ring (Figure 7). To measure D_{ab} or D_{bc} in the vinyl group it is necessary to measure the observed split tings in the vinyl group as a function of H_0^2, extrapolating to zero field strength to obtain J_{ab} or J_{bc}, and obtaining D_{ab} or D_{bc} at 600 MHz from the slope of the plot.

Table 3 gives the observed splittings at several field strengths, from which we obtain D_{bc} = − 0.295 Hz at 600 MHz in the Zn–complex, and −0.389 Hz at 600 MHz for 0.01M solution in C^2HCl_3. The proportions to the CH_2 splittings are exactly equal: D_{bc}/D_{CH_2} = − 0.22, and we conclude that the geometry is not particularly affected by dimer formation. From equation 17 we deduce that

$$\frac{D_{bc}}{D_{CH_2}} = \frac{(1/2) <3 \cos^2\alpha_{bc} - 1>}{(1/2) <3 \cos^2\alpha_{CH_2} - 1>} \frac{a_{CH_2}^3}{a_{bc}^3} \qquad [20]$$

All members of this are well known except $1/2 <3\cos^2\alpha_{bc}-1>$, which is calculated to be −0.251. From solid geometry,

$$\cos\alpha_{bc} = \sin\theta \sin\phi \qquad [21]$$

where ϕ is the angle between the internuclear axis bc and the rotation axis R, taken as 31.5°. Solution provides ϕ = ±51°, so that the vinyl group is demonstrated to be strongly twisted out of the porphyrin plane. The changes in splitting for H_aH_b and H_aH_c are much smaller, because of the a^3 dependence, so the determination of α is subject to large errors. However, it is confirmatory evidence that the geometry deduced here leads to the prediction that the H_aH_b splitting will decrease and that the H_aH_c splitting will increase with higher field strength, roughly as observed.

This appears to be a generally applicable method for the investigation of aggregation and molecular geometry in solution, with obvious application to nucleic acid helices. The effects, even at 600 MHz, are small and require careful and painstaking measurement, but are nevertheless quite exactly interpretable. Since the effects increase as the square of the field strength, advances to yet higher fields will cause the effects to be very conspicuous in many cases.

The two topics reported on above are partial results of more extensive collaborative programs with able and hard–working colleagues to whom I am greatly indebted. In the development of the CAMELSPIN experiment, Miss Ju–mee Lee, Dr. Richard Stephens, Dr. P.K. Mishra, and Dr. Donald Davis played important parts. The investigation of the erythronolide A derivatives was stimulated by the late Prof. K. Sakan, and his student S. Babirad. In the exploration of field–induced orientation phenomena, Dr. C. Gayathri, Mr. Peter C. M. van Zijl, Dr. Peter Domaille, and Prof. C. MacLean are valued partners. Professor K. Smith has supplied the porphyrins for study. I also especially thank my colleague, Josef

Dadok, for the instrumentation design and nurture which made the work possible. Financial support was provided by grants RR00292 and AM16532 from the National Institutes of Health and CHE8206281 from the National Science Foundation.

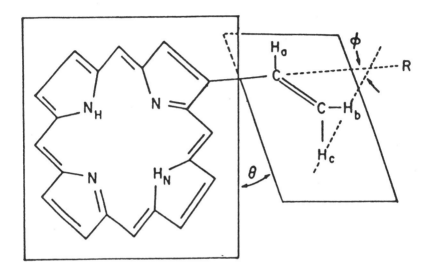

FIG. 7. Rotation of vinyl group relative to porphyrin ring.

Table 3. Splittings in the Vinyl Proton Signals of Vinylphylloerythrin Methyl Ester at Various Field Strengths

Sample	Splitting	Observed Separation		
		5.875 T	11.75 T	14.09 T
Free porphyrin in C^2HCl_3	$J_{bc}+D_{bc}$	1.79 Hz	1.58 Hz	1.47 Hz
	$J_{ab}+D_{ab}$	11.50 Hz	11.46 Hz	11.40 Hz
	$J_{ac}+D_{ac}$	17.79 Hz	17.80 Hz	17.85 Hz
Zn complex in $C_5^2H_5N$	$J_{bc}+D_{bc}$	1.81 Hz	1.64 Hz	1.57 Hz
	$J_{ab}+D_{ab}$	11.56 Hz	11.52 Hz	11.46 Hz
	$J_{ac}+D_{ac}$	17.83 Hz	17.77 Hz	17.77 Hz

REFERENCES

1. Abraham, R.J., Eivazi, F., Nayyir–Mazhir, R., Pearson, H., and Smith, K.M. (1978): Org. Magn. Res. 11:52–54.
2. Battaglia, M.R. and Ritchie, G.L.D. (1977): J. Chem. Soc. Faraday Trans. 2, 73:209–221.
3. Bothner–By, A.A. (1979): In: Biological Applications of Magnetic Resonance, edited by R. Shulman, pp. 177–219. Academic Press, New York.
4. Chou, S.H., Hare, D.R., Wemmer, D.E., and Reid, B.R. (1983): Biochemistry 22:3037–3041.
5. Closs, G.L., Katz, J.J., Pennington, F.C., Thomas, M.R., and Strain, H.H. (1963): J. Am. Chem. Soc. 85:3809–3821.
6. Emsley, J.W. and Lindon, J.C. (1975): In: NMR Spectroscopy Using Liquid Crystal Solvents. Pergamon Press, New York.
7. Flygare, W.H. (1974): Chem. Rev. 74:653–687.
8. Gayathri, C., Bothner–By, A.A., van Zijl, P.C.M., and MacLean, C. (1982): Phys. Letters 87:192–196.
9. Kalk, A. and Berendson, H.J.C. (1976): J. Magn. Reson. 24:343–366.
10. Keller, R.M. and Wüthrich, K. (1980): Biochem. Biophys. Acta, 621:204–217.
11. Lohman, J.A.B. and MacLean, C. (1978): Phys. Letters 58:483–486.
12. Lonsdale, K. and Krishnan, K.S. (1936): Proc. Roy. Soc. A156:597–613.
13. Macura, S. and Ernst, R.R. (1980): Mol. Phys. 41:95–117; Macura, S., Huang, Y., Smith, D., and Ernst, R.R. (1981):J. Magn. Reson. 43:259–281.
14. Maier, W. and Saupe, A. (1958): Z. Naturforch 13A:564–566; Maier, W. and Saupe, A. (1960): Z. Naturforch 15A:287–292.
15. Masamune, S., Bates, G.S., and Corcoran, J.W. (1977): Angew. Chem. Int. Ed. Engl. 16:585–607.
16. Nicolaou, K.C. (1977): Tetrahedron 33:683–710.
17. Noggle, J.H. and Schirmer, R.F. (1971): The Nuclear Overhauser Effect, Academic Press, New York.
18. Pople, J.A., Schneider, W.G., and Bernstein, H.J. (1959): In: High Resolution Nuclear Magnetic Resonance. McGraw–Hill, New York.
19. Solomon, I. (1955): Phys. Rev., 99:559–565.
20. Williamson, M.P. (1983): J. Magn. Reson. 55:471–479.
21. Woodward, R.B., Logusch, E., Nambiar, K.P., Sakan, K., Ward, D.E., Au–Yeung, B.–W., Balaram, P., Browne, L.J., Card, P.J., Chen, C.H., Chenevert, R.B., Fliri, A., Fribel, K., Gais, H.–J., Garratt, D.G., Hayakawa, K., Heggie, W., Hesson, D.P., Hoppe, D., Hoppe, I., Hyatt, J.A., Ikeda, D., Jacobi, P.A., Kim, K.S., Kobuke, Y., Kojima, K., Krowicki, K.A, Lee, V.J., Leutert, T., Malchenko, S., Martens, J., Matthews, R.S., Ong, B.S., Press, J.B., Babu, T.V. Rajan, Rousseau, G., Sauter, H.M.. Suzuki, M., Tatsuta, K., Tolbert, L.M., Truesdale, E.A., Uchida, I., Ueda, Y., Uyehara, T., Vasella, A.T., Vladuchick, W.C., Wade, P.A., Williams, R.M., and Wong, H.N.–C. (1982): J. Am. Chem. Soc. 103:3210–3213, 3213–3215, 3215–3217.
22. van Zijl, P.C.M., Ruessink, B.H., Bulthuis, J., and MacLean, C. (1984): Accts. Chem. Res. 17:172–180.

NMR in Biology and Medicine,
edited by Shu Chien and Chien Ho.
Raven Press, New York © 1986.

Interaction of Polypeptide Antibiotics with Phospholipid Bilayers: A ^{31}P and ^{2}H NMR Study*

Raphael Zidovetzki **, Utpal Banerjee, Robert R. Birge, †
and Sunney I. Chan

Arthur Amos Noyes Laboratory of Chemical Physics, California Institute of Technology, Pasadena, California 91125

INTRODUCTION

In recent years, there has been considerable interest in the mechanism of action of polypeptide antibiotics. The biological activity of some of these antibiotics is thought to be due to their amphipathic character which would enable the molecules to interact with (and presumably disrupt) the outer cell membrane of gram–negative bacteria. We report here studies aimed at clarifying the molecular details of interactions of four poly-peptide antibiotics with bilayer membranes: polymyxin B, gramicidin S, valinomycin, and alamethicin.

Polymyxin B sulfate is a cyclic polypeptide containing five positively charged diamino–butyric acid residues (21). Lipid–polymyxin B interactions have been studied using a variety of biophysical methods, including fluorescence polarization, electron microscopy (6), electron paramagnetic resonance spectroscopy (4), calorimetry (20), and Raman spectroscopy (15). Some data suggest that polymyxin B does not interact with zwitterionic lipids (6,23), while others implicate that polymyxin B interacts with such lipids (15).

Gramicidin S is a cyclodecapeptide antibiotic isolated from Bacillus grevis (5), also effective against gram–negative bacteria. It was suggested that the action of gramicidin S involves interactions with negatively charged lipids (2,8). Following initial adsorption on the membrane surface via the ionic interactions, it has been suggested that the hydrophobic residues of gramicidin S can also come in contact with the acyl side chains of the lipids (24).

---

* Contribution No. 7364 from Arthur Amos Noyes Laboratory of Chemical Physics, California Institute of Technology, Pasadena, CA 91125.

** Present address: Department of Biology, University of California, Riverside, CA 92521.

† Present address: Department of Chemistry, Carnegie–Mellon University, Pittsburgh, PA 15213.

Valinomycin is a cyclododecadepsipeptide antibiotic produced by Streptomyces fulvissimus. Valinomycin alters the ionic permeability of natural (14) and artificial (13) lipid membranes. Previous studies using ^{1}H–NMR (7) and Raman spectroscopy (22) have provided evidence that valinomycin can penetrate into the bilayers of dimyristoyl lecithin (DML), but apparently this incorporation of the peptide into the bilayer membrane is not accompanied by any disruption of the ordering of the lipid chains.

Alamethicin is an icosapeptide extruded from the fungus Trichoderma viride which exhibits voltage–gated ionic conductance in black lipid films (10). There has been debate in the literature about the partitioning of this peptide into the bilayer membrane. Some studies have argued that alamethicin is primarily a surface active molecule with minimal partitioning of the peptide into the hydrophobic part of the membrane, particularly in the absence of an electric field (11,12), while others have proposed complete partitioning of alamethicin into bilayer membranes (3,10).

In this work, we have compared the interactions of these four antibiotics with various lipid bilayers: (i) a multilamellar dispersion of DML; and (ii) a mixture of phospholipids similar in lipid composition to that of outer cell membrane of gram–negative bacteria (model E. coli membranes). Two NMR probes located in different parts of the bilayer membranes have been exploited: ^{31}P NMR of the phosphorus moiety of the lipid headgroups provides information on perturbation by the peptide near the aqueous–bilayer interface; ^{2}H NMR of deuterated lipid chains was used to monitor the orientational order of the hydrophobic region. The results obtained showed that only gramicidin S disrupted the organization of DML bilayers. Alamethicin and valinomycin were shown to interact with the bilayers at the aqueous–membrane interface only. No significant interaction was observed between DML bilayers and polymyxin B.

In contrast, all the antibiotic molecules interacted strongly with the model E. coli membranes. ^{2}H–NMR showed that the phosphatidyl-ethanolamine (PE) and phosphatidylglycerol (PG) components of the model E. coli membranes are involved.

MATERIALS AND METHODS

Dimyristoyl phosphatidylcholine (DML) was obtained from Sigma (St. Louis, MO) and was checked for purity by thin layer chromatography. All other unlabelled synthetic lipids [dipalmitoylphosphatidylethanolamine (DPPE) and dipalmitoylphosphatidylglycerol (DPPG)] and all ^{2}H–labelled lipids [diperdeuteromyristoylphosphatidylcholine (DML–d_{54}); diperdeutero-palmitoylphosphatidylethanolamine (DPPE–d_{62}) and diperdeuteropalmitoyl-phosphatidylglycerol (DPPG–d_{62})] were purchased from Avanti Polar Lipids, Birmingham, AL, and were shown to be pure by thin layer chromatography. Unlabelled lipid extracts from E. coli cell membrane: phosphatidylethanolamine (PE) and diphosphatidylglycerol (DPG, cardiolipin) were also obtained from Avanti Polar Lipids.

Gramicidin S dihydrochloride (Sigma) was dissolved in H_2O–dioxane (5:2 v/v), filtered and lyophilized prior to use. Polymyxin B sulfate was from Sigma. Valinomycin was purchased from Calbiochem (San Diego, CA).

Multilamellar dispersions of the various lipids used in this study were prepared as follows. First, the lipids, or the lipid–antibiotic mixture, were dissolved in methanol or $CHCl_3$ in an NMR tube. The solvent was then evaporated off with dry nitrogen, and the tube was kept under vacuum for at least eight hours. The thin film thus formed was hydrated with a 25 mM Tris buffer solution (pD 7.4) in D_2O by repeated vortexing on a mixer and gentle warming with a heat gun. The vortexing was continued for about five minutes until a uniform white suspension was obtained. The samples were always fully hydrated and was typically 1:10 w/v in lipid to water. In the experiments with polymyxin B, the antibiotic was added to the dry lipids as a solution in the TRIS buffer. Model E. coli membranes, i.e., multilayers with composition similar to the E. coli membranes, consisted of 59% PE, 19% DPPE, 19% DPPG and 3% DPG. In the ^{2}H–NMR experiments, either DPPE or DPPG was substituted with DPPE–d_{62} or DPPG–d_{62}, respectively.

^{31}P– and ^{2}H–NMR spectra were acquired at 11.74T (500.13 MHz ^{1}H frequency) on a Bruker WM500 spectrometer as previously described (1).

RESULTS AND DISCUSSION

Studies with DML Bilayers

^{31}P–NMR Study of Interactions of the Antibiotics with DML. Typical ^{31}P–NMR spectra of DML multilayers with and without added antibiotics are given in Figure 1. The ^{31}P spectrum of the control DML sample is characteristic of the lipid molecules in the bilayer phase (18). The rapid intramolecular isomerization of the head–group and the rotational diffusion of the lipid molecules about an axis perpendicular to the plane of the bilayer (director) causes axial averaging. Only two components of the axially averaged chemical shift tensor (σ) can be obtained, corresponding to the parallel ($\sigma_{\}}$) or perpendicular ($\sigma_{\perp}$) orientations relative to the director. The chemical shift anisotropy $\Delta\sigma = \sigma_{\}} - \sigma_{\perp}$, can be determined from the splitting between the edges of the spectrum at the half height of the low–frequency "foot" (Figure 1). This spectral parameter depends on the molecular motions averaging the chemical shift interactions, as well as the average orientation of the phospholipid headgroups relative to the director. As the motional state of the lipids depends on temperature, and, in particular, undergoes an abrupt change at the gel–liquid crystalline phase transition temperature (T_c) of the lipid, $\Delta\sigma$ offers a useful handle to monitor the effect of each of the antibiotics on the phase transition temperature and to compare the motional state of DML in the absence and presence of the antibiotics.

^{31}P–NMR spectra of the DML–antibiotic mixtures (Figure 1B–D) all showed the same spectral pattern characteristic of the multilamellar bilayer state (Figure 1A). Thus, even at the antibiotic:DML molar ratio of 1:5.7, the bilayer phase is still maintained in the presence of these antibiotics. Disruption of bilayer structure was observed only in the case of gramicidin S with further increase of the antibiotic concentration.

The ^{31}P–NMR spectra of DML multilayers in the presence of different concentrations of alamethicin are depicted in Figure 2. The bilayer phase of DML is maintained even in the presence of alamethicin:DML molar ratio of 1:2.

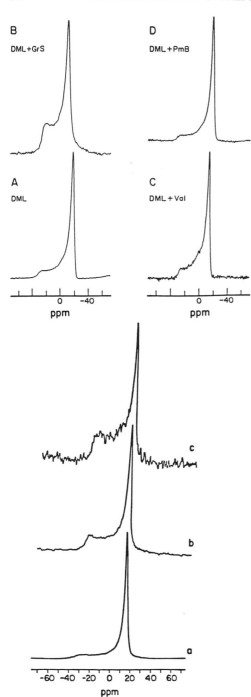

FIG. 1 ^{31}P–NMR spectra of lipid headgroups in fully hydrated DML–antibiotic mixtures. The spectra were recorded at 202.49 MHz frequency at 25.3°C. The composition of the samples with antibiotics was 1:5.7 (antibiotic:DML molar ratio). (A) DML, (B) DML plus gramicidin S, (C) DML plus valinomycin, (D) DML plus polymyxin B.

FIG. 2 ^{31}P–NMR spectra of lipid headgroups in fully hydrated DML–alamethicin mixtures. The spectra were recorded at 2.249–MHz at 26°C. (a) DML, (b) 1:15 alamethicin: DML molar ratio, (c) 1:2 alamethicin: DML molar ratio.

Figures 3–6 summarize the temperature dependence of $\Delta\sigma$ for DML in the presence of different concentrations of antibiotics. The effects of the antibiotic on $\Delta\sigma$ are clearly different in each case.

In the case of polymyxin B (Figure 3) the presence of the antibiotic does not change the values of $\Delta\sigma$ either above or below the phase transition temperature. This is true even at the polymyxin B:lipid molar ratio of 1:5.7. Only at a higher concentration of polymyxin B (1:3) was a small (4°) change in the phase transition temperature of the DML noted. These results are consistent with earlier studies which showed that polymyxin B does not interact with neutral lipids (23).

The effects of valinomycin on the $\Delta\sigma$ of DML are shown in Figure 4. Above T_c, we noted that $\Delta\sigma$ is <u>decreased</u> in the presence of valinomycin at molar ratios of valinomycin to DML of both 1:16 and 1:5.5. The phase transition temperature is also decreased by 5° in the presence of the antibiotic. These results indicate that valinomycin, unlike polymyxin B, does interact with DML bilayers.

The effect of gramicidin S on the $\Delta\sigma$ of DML is again quite different (Figure 5). While the effect of the antibiotic on the bilayer at a gramicidin S:DML molar ratio of 1:33 is negligible (Figure 5), increasing the concentration of gramicidin S to the molar ratios of 1:16 and 1:5.5 does result in significant changes in $\Delta\sigma$. The perturbation seems to be most pronounced <u>in the</u> <u>vicinity</u> of the phase transition temperature (Figure 5). At a molar ratio of 1:16, gramicidin S depresses the thermal phase transition temperature of DML by 3° and affects the values of $\Delta\sigma$ within a narrow range of temperatures (about 3°C) immediately above T_c. The perturbation of the bilayer becomes even more prominent when the gramicidin S concentration is increased to a molar ratio of 1:5.5. The phase transition temperature of DML is now decreased by 6°C, and $\Delta\sigma$ is affected within a range of temperature of 10° immediately above the T_c, decreasing monotonously with decreasing temperature and reaching a minimum of 36 ppm at 18°C, just above the thermal phase transition temperature (Figure 5). A careful examination of the ^{31}P spectra for the gramicidin S–DML systems reveals additional complications. In the vicinity of T_c at a gramicidin S:DML molar ratio of 1:16, the spectra obtained at 19° and 17.4°C (Figure 7, right) appear to be weighted superpositions of the spectra obtained above T_c, at 27°C, and below T_c, at 14.2°C (Figure 7, right). This observation is consistent with the coexistence of both gel and liquid crystalline phases. Such phase separation was not observed by us for the other antibiotics studied. As further evidence of the interaction of gramicidin S with DML bilayers, we note that ^{31}P-NMR lineshape degenerates into a single resonance position characteristic of isotropic motions of the phospholipid molecules when the antibiotic concentration is increased to 1:2.7. This observation suggests disruption of the bilayer and solubilization of the lipid by the antibiotic to give small vesicles or micelles. In contrast, even at this concentration of gramicidin S, $\Delta\sigma$ is not affected by the presence of the antibiotic below T_c. For example, the ^{31}P-NMR lineshape obtained when the dispersion is cooled to 13.5°C suggests the re-formation of bilayers. At 9.5°C, the bulk of the intensity of the ^{31}P-spectra is associated with the bilayer powder pattern (Figure 8, right).

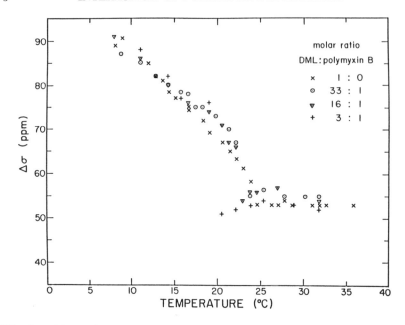

FIG. 3 Plot of Δσ vs. temperature for polymyxin B–containing DML multilayers. (x——x) no polymyxin B; (o——o) 1:33 polymyxin B: DML molar ratio; (∇——∇) 1:16 polymyxin B: DML molar ratio; (+——+) 1:3 polymyxin B: DML molar ratio.

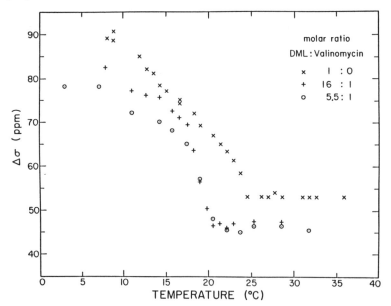

FIG. 4 Plot of Δσ vs. temperature for valinomycin–containing DML multilayers. (x——x) no valinomycin; (+——+) 1:16 valinomycin: DML molar ratio; (o——o) 1:5.5 valinomycin: DML molar ratio.

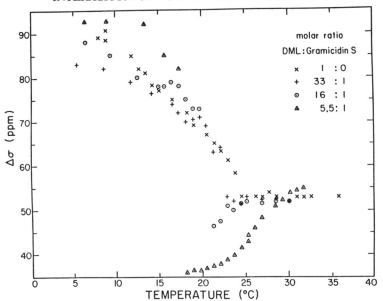

FIG. 5   Plot of Δσ vs. temperature for gramicidin S–containing DML multilayers. (x——x) no gramicidin S; (+——+) 1:33 gramicidin S: DML molar ratio; (o——o) 1:16 gramicidin S: DML molar ratio; (Δ——Δ) 1:5.5 gramicidin S: DML molar ratio.

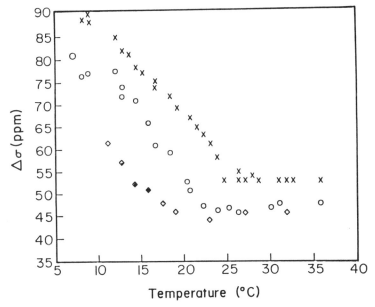

FIG. 6   The effect of alamethicin on the ^{31}P chemical shift anisotropy of the lipid phosphorus on DML multilayers at various temperatures. (x——x) no alamethicin added; (o——o) 1:15 alamethicin: DML molar ratio; (◊——◊) 1:2 alamethicin: DML molar ratio.

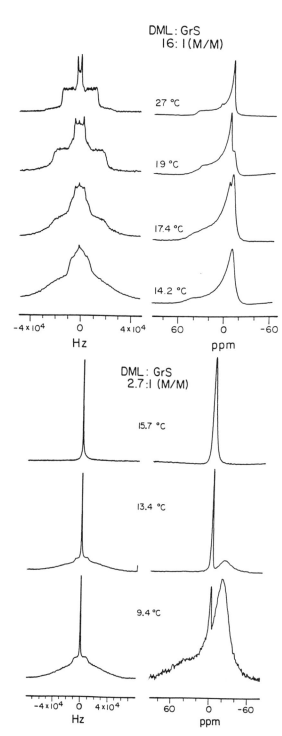

FIG. 7 ^{31}P– (right) and ^{2}H– (left) NMR spectra of DML with added gramicidin S at different temperatures. The gramicidin S: DML molar ratio was 1:16.

FIG. 8 ^{31}P– (right) and ^{2}H– (left) NMR spectra with added gramicidin S at different temperatures. The gramidicin S: DML molar ratio was 1:2.7.

Figure 6 summarizes the temperature dependence of $\Delta\sigma$ for DML multilayers in the presence of alamethicin. The phase transition temperature of DML is only decreased slightly (about 2°) in the presence of alamethicin, even at the molar ratio of 1:15 for the antibiotic. Further increase in the alamethicin concentration to the molar ratio of 1:2 suppresses T_C by 4°. Throughout the range of temperatures studied, the presence of alamethicin resulted in the decrease of $\Delta\sigma$. Above T_C, the perturbation of the bilayer headgroups as evidenced by ^{31}P NMR was already saturated at the alamethicin:lipid molar ratio of 1:15.

We have performed extensive simulations of the ^{31}P NMR lineshape in order to ascertain those motional parameters that can account for the observed change of $\Delta\sigma$ (1). From these results we attribute the observed decrease of $\Delta\sigma$ for alamethicin–, valinomycin–, and gramicidin S–containing bilayers to changes in the tilt angles ϕ and θ of the phospholipid headgroups relative to the director. In the case of alamethicin and valinomycin, this change in tilt angles is temperature independent above T_C (Figures 4 and 6). In the case of gramicidin S, however, the changes in tilt angles are temperature dependent above T_C, with the most pronounced effect immediately above the phase transition temperature (Figure 5).

^{2}H–NMR Studies of Interactions of the Antibiotics with DML. Further information on interaction of the antibiotics with DML was deduced from ^{2}H–NMR studies of chain perdeuterated DML. The ^{2}H–NMR spectra of DML–d_{54} at several temperatures above the thermal phase transition of the lipid are shown on Figure 9. Each of these spectra represents the superposition of axially averaged powder patterns arising from the different deuterons for the various CD_2 segments along the acyl chains. The CD bond order parameter for the ith segment, S_{CD}, can be derived from the quadrupolar splitting observed at the perpendicular orientation, $\Delta\nu$, using the relation

$$\Delta\nu_D^i = \left(\frac{3}{4}\right)(e^2qQ/h)\ S_{CD}^i \ ,$$

where (e^2qQ/h) is the CD deuteron quadrupolar coupling constant. It has been shown by specific deuteration of lipids that there is an order parameter profile along the hydrocarbon chains of a phospholipid molecule in a multilayer, with a characteristic plateau for those methylene segments near the glycerol backbone (17). The corresponding quadrupolar patterns due to these segments are nearly coincident with one another, and the signals at the perpendicular orientations overlap near the edge of the spectrum. Since the lower parts of the chains are more disordered, the quadrupolar patterns from these methylene segments show well–resolved peaks at the perpendicular orientation. Above T_C, up to thirteen quadrupolar splittings can be discerned for DML–d_{54} (1).

We have examined the effect of the various antibiotics under study here on the quadrupolar splittings of DML over the same range of temperatures and antibiotic concentrations used in the ^{31}P–NMR measurements. The ^{2}H–NMR spectra of DML–d_{54} in the presence of each of the antibiotics studied are given in Figures 10 and 11.

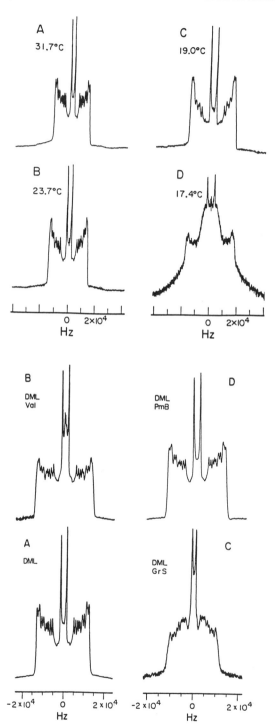

FIG. 9 ^{2}H–NMR spectra of DML–d$_{54}$ multilayers at different temperatures.

FIG. 10 ^{2}H–NMR spectra of DML–d$_{54}$ multilayers with added antibiotics at 32°C. (A) no antibiotic added; (B) with valinomycin; (C) with gramidicin S; (D) with polymyxin B. The antibiotic: lipid molar ratio was 1:5.7 in (B), (C) and (D).

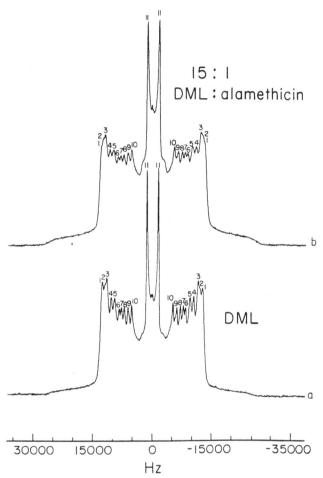

FIG. 11 ^{2}H–NMR spectra of DML multilayer with perdeuterated hydrocarbon chains. (a) DML–d_{54} only. (b) 1:15 alamethicin: DML–d_{54} molar ratio. Tentative assigments of peaks 1 through 11 are given in Banerjee et al. (1).

A comparison of the spectra in the presence (Figure 10D) and absence (Figure 10A) of polymyxin B shows that this antibiotic has no effect on the hydrocarbon chains of the bilayer. Based on these observations, together with ^{31}P NMR results described earlier (Figures 1 and 3), we can conclude that polymyxin B does not interact with DML.

A slightly different picture emerges in the case of valinomycin. The ^{2}H–spectra of DML–d_{54} in the presence of valinomycin reveal some small effects of this antibiotic on the hydrocarbon chains (Figure 10B). A small change in the quadrupolar splitting is observed for the outermost peak arising from the methylene segments near the glycerol backbone; however, all the other splittings remain unchanged. The spectrum with valinomycin also does not show spectral broadening typically observed upon the incorporation of membrane proteins into bilayers (16,19). These observations of the effects of valinomycin on the ^{31}P- and ^{2}H–NMR spectra of DML are consistent with the antibiotic molecule interacting primarily with the headgroups of the lipids near the bilayer–water interface.

Figure 11 compares the ^{2}H–NMR spectrum of DML-d_{54} above the phase transition in the absence and presence of alamethicin. As in the case of valinomycin, the presence of alamethicin has only minimal effect on the hydrocarbon chains of the bilayer, specifically, in the outermost peak arising from the methylene segments near the glycerol backbone. The remaining peaks all stay unchanged in the presence of alamethicin (Figure 11). Thus, as in the case of valinomycin, ^{2}H–and ^{31}P–NMR show that alamethicin interacts only with the headgroups of the DML bilayer membrane.

The ^{2}H–NMR spectrum of DML-d_{54} in the presence of gramicidin S is given in Figure 10C. The addition of gramidicin S results in both the broadening of the DML spectrum and changes in the spectral shape. These results, together with the ^{31}P–NMR measurements mentioned earlier, indicate that gramicidin S does disrupt the bilayer membrane above the phase transistion temperature. However, the phase behavior seems quite complex, as noted by ^{31}P–NMR (Figures 7,8 right) and ^{2}H–NMR (Figures 7,8 left). In the vicinity of the phase transistion temperature both ^{31}P– and ^{2}H–NMR indicate the coexistence of liquid crystalline and gel phases at gramcidin S: DML molar ratio of 1:16 (Figure 7). Increasing the gramicidin S concentration to antibiotic: DML molar ratio of 1:2.7 in fact causes complete disruption of the bilayer. However, even in this case, bilayers are re–formed upon cooling of the sample (Figure 8).

Studies with Model E. coli Membranes

The biological activity of polymyxin B and gramicidin S is directed against the outer cell membrane of gram–negative bacteria, which is rich in other phospholipids, i.e. PE and PG. Accordingly we have attempted to mimic the E. coli outer membrane using a mixture of E. coli lipid extracts and synthetic lipids (see Methods), to construct bilayers with a composition similar to the composition of the outer cell membrane of E. coli, and have examined the interaction of such bilayers with the antibiotics using ^{31}P– and ^{2}H–NMR.

^{31}P–NMR Studies Using Model E. coli Membranes. The ^{31}P spectra of the multilayers in the absence and presence of the various antibiotics are presented in Figure 12. These spectral results of the fully hydrated lipids indicate that the lipids are principally in bilayer conformation (Figure 12A). However, with each of the three antibiotics studied, a peak at a position corresponding to fast and isotropic motionally averaged phospholipids is also observed. This indicates that the antibiotics induce to various degrees the formation of lipid micelles or small vesicles, even at antibiotic: lipid molar ratio of 1:16. This effect is the smallest in the case of polymyxin B, with only a minor portion of the intensity of the signal being in the isotropic peak (Figure 12C). The isotropic peak becomes more prominent in the case of added valinomycin (Figure 12B), and becomes dominant in the presence of gramicidin S (Figure 12D).

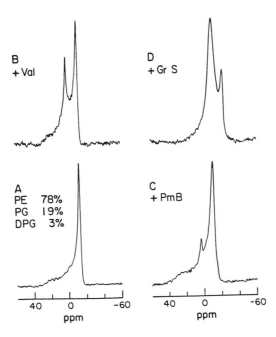

FIG. 12 ^{31}P–NMR spectra of lipid headgroups of model E. coli membranes (see text) with added antibiotics at 25.3°C. The composition of the samples with antibiotic was 1:16 antibiotic: lipid molar ratio: (A) no antibiotics added; (B) with valinomycin; (C) with polymyxin B; (D) with gramicidin S.

^{2}H–NMR Studies Using Model E. coli Membranes. In order to further characterize the interaction of the antibiotics with model E. coli membranes, we substituted part of the lipids with synthetic lipids containing perdeuterated side chains. In one study we substituted DPPG with DPPG–d_{62}, and in another we substituted 25% of E. coli PE extract with synthetic DPPE–d_{62}. The ^{2}H–NMR spectrum of DPPE–d_{62} (Figure 13A) is similar to the spectrum of DPPG–d_{62} (Figure 13B) in chemically identical model E. coli membranes.

The ^{2}H–spectra of both PE and PG are significantly altered upon the addition of polymyxin B at a molar ratio of 1:16 (Figure 14). The shapes of both spectra are still characteristic of the bilayer conformation, with only a small portion of intensity being in the isotropic peak in the center, consistent with the ^{31}P–NMR results noted earlier (Figure 12C). These spectra, however, exhibit line broadening, which obscures the fine structure typically observed for pure lipids (Figure 13). Both the broadening effect and the intensity of the isotropic peak are somewhat more pronounced in the spectrum of DPPE–d_{62} (Figure 14B), probably indicating that polymyxin B interacts more strongly with the PE than with PG.

CONTROL; 78% PE; 19% PG; 3% DPG

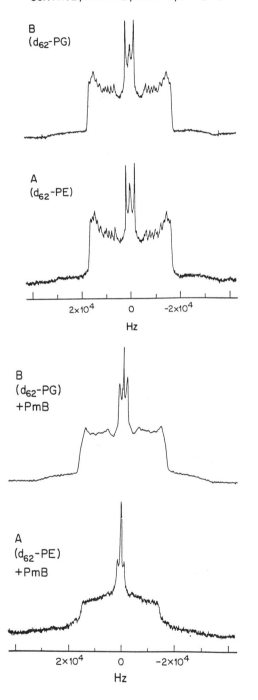

FIG. 13 ^{2}H–NMR spectra of ^{2}H–labelled lipids in model E. coli membranes. (A) DPPE–d$_{62}$; (B) DPPG–d$_{62}$.

FIG. 14 ^{2}H–NMR spectra of deuterated lipids in model E. coli membranes with added polymyxin B at 32°C. Polymyxin B: lipid molar ratio was 1:5.7. (A) ^{2}H–labelled PE; (B) ^{2}H–labelled PG.

The preferential interaction of the antibiotic with the PE component of the membrane is more pronounced in the case of gramicidin S (Figure 15). The ^{2}H–spectrum of DPPG–d$_{62}$ in the presence of gramicidin S still has most of the intensity in the bilayer shape (Figure 15B). It does exhibit line broadening similar to the one observed in the case of polymyxin B. The bilayer structure is maintained, however, only by a small percentage of the PE component, most of this lipid giving the isotropic ^{2}H–NMR peak (Figure 15A). Since the PE comprises 78% of model bilayers, and the PG only 19%, the isotropic peak of the ^{31}P–spectrum of the lipids with gramicidin S can be attributed to PE, while the bilayer part of the spectrum to both the PG and the part of the PE.

The ^{2}H–spectrum of DPPE–d$_{62}$ in the model E. coli membrane in the presence of valinomycin is given in Figure 16. As in the case of gramicidin S, valinomycin also significantly disrupts the bilayer structure.

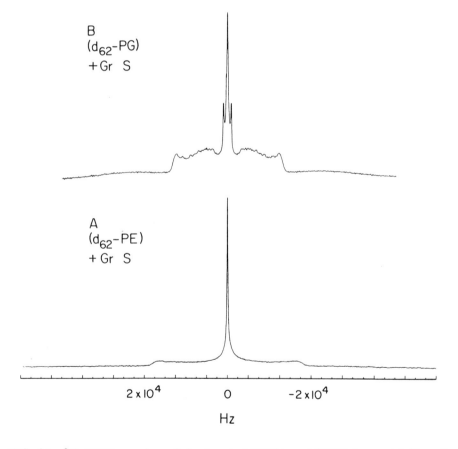

FIG. 15 ^{2}H–NMR spectra of deuterated PE(A) and PG(B) in model E. coli membranes with added gramicidin S at 32°C. Gramicidin S: lipid molar ratio was 1:5.7.

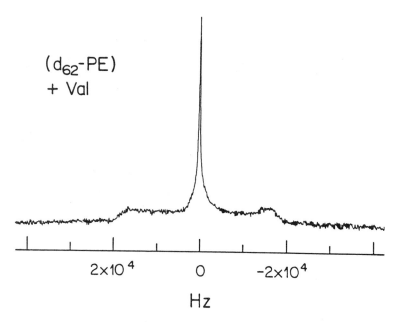

FIG. 16 ^{2}H–NMR spectra of deuterated PE in model $\underline{E}$. $\underline{coli}$ membranes with added valinomycin at 32°C. Valinomycin: lipid molar ratio was 1:5.7.

CONCLUSIONS

We have shown in this preliminary report how the combined use of ^{31}P–NMR of the lipid headgroups and ^{2}H–NMR of the acyl side chains can be used to probe the interaction of peptide antibiotics with the lipid membranes. With the peptide antibiotics selected for this study, we have concluded that polymyxin B does not interact with DML, and that valinomycin and alamethicin interact with surface of DML bilayers at the aqueous bilayer interface only. Unlike the other two antibiotics, gramicidin S perturbs the structure of the bilayer at both phospholipid headgroups and the acyl side chains, provided that the antibiotic concentration is sufficiently high; thus, this antibiotic does penetrate the DML bilayer. These interactions take place, however, only above the phase transition temperature of the lipids.

A completely different picture emerges from the studies with the model $\underline{E}$. $\underline{coli}$ bilayers containing typical concentrations of PE and PG. Here, we have obtained evidence for insertion of polymyxin B molecule into the bilayer membrane without disrupting it. Both valinomycin and gramicidin S, however, exhibit strong destructive effects on the model $\underline{E}$. $\underline{coli}$ membranes. In the case of gramicidin S, a preferential interaction with the PE component was noted. The interaction of valinomycin with the PE is also very strong. The interaction of each of these antibiotics with PE is probably one of the sources of their toxicity, as PE is one of the major components of the mammalian cell membranes.

ACKNOWLEDGMENTS

This research was supported by Grant GM–22432 from the National Institute of General Medical Sciences, U.S. Public Health Service. The Southern California Regional NMR facility is funded by Grants CHE–7916324 and CHE–8440137 from the National Science Foundation.

REFERENCES

1. Banerjee, U., Zidovetzki, R., Birge, R.R., and Chan, S.I. (1985): Biochemistry 24:7621–7627.
2. Eremin, V., Sepetov, N.F., Sibelbina, L.A., Lorbkipanidze, A.E., and Ostrovskii, D.N. (1979): Dokl. Akad. Nauk, USSR 245:994–997.
3. Fringeli, U.P. and Fringeli, M. (1979): Proc. Natl. Acad. Sci. USA 76:3852–3856.
4. Galla, H.J. and Trudell, J.R. (1980): Biochim. Biophys. Acta 602:522–530.
5. Gause, G.F. and Brazhnikova, M.G. (1944): Nature 154:703.
6. Hartman, W., Galla, H.J., and Sackmann, E. (1978): Biochim. Biophys. Acta 510:129–139.
7. Hsu, M.C. and Chan, S.I. (1973): Biochemistry 12:3872–3876.
8. Ishida, M. and Mizushima, J.S. (1969): J. Biochem. 66:33–43.
9. Latorre, R. and Alvarez, D. (1981): Physiol. Rev. 61:71–150.
10. Latorre, R., Miller, C.G., and Quay, S. (1981): Biophys. J. 36:803–809.
11. Lau, A.L.Y. and Chan, S.I. (1975): Proc. Natl. Acad. Sci. USA 72:2170–2174.
12. Lau, A.L.Y. and Chan, S.I. (1976): Biochemistry 15:2551–2555.
13. Lev, A.A. and Buzhinsky, E.P. (1967): Tsitologiya 9:102–106.
14. Moore, C. and Pressman, B.C. (1964): Biochem. Biophys. Res. Commun. 15:562–567.
15. Mushayakarara, E. and Levin, I.W. (1984): Biochim. Biophys. Acta 769:585–595.
16. Rice, D.M. Hsung, J.C. King, G.E., and Oldfield, E. (1979):. J. Am. Chem. Soc. 18:5885–5892.
17. Seelig, J. (1977): Quart. Rev. Biophys. 10:353–418.
18. Seelig, J. (1978): Biochim. Biophys. Acta 515:105–140.
19. Seelig, A. and Seelig, J. (1978): Hoppe–Seyler's Z. Physiol. Chem. 359:1747–1756.
20. Sixl, F. and Galla, H.J. (1982): Biochim. Biophys. Acta 633:466–478.
21. Storm, D.R., Rosenthal, K.S., and Swanson, P.E. (1977): Ann. Rev. Biochem. 46:723–763.
22. Susi, H., Sampugna, J., Hampson, J.W., and Ard, J.S. (1979): Biochemistry 18:297–301.
23. Teuber, M. and Miller, I.R. (1977): Biochim. Biophys. Acta 467:280–289.
24. Yonezawa, H., Okamoto, K., Kaneda, M., Tominaga, N., and Izumiya, N. (1982): 20th Symposium on Peptide Chemistry, Tojonako, Japan, pp. 283–288.

NMR in Biology and Medicine,
edited by Shu Chien and Chien Ho.
Raven Press, New York © 1986.

Nuclear Magnetic Resonance Studies of Nucleic Acids

Lou–sing Kan and Paul O.P. Ts'o

*Division of Biophysics, School of Hygiene and Public Health, Johns Hopkins University,
Baltimore, Maryland 21205*

The genetic materials, deoxyribonucleic acid (DNA) and ribonucleic acid (RNA) are the cornerstones of life. However, the composition of DNA or RNA is much simpler than that of proteins, which contain 20 different amino acids. Nucleic acids consist of three molecular fragments: sugar, heterocylic bases and phosphate. The sugar is a cyclic furanoside ribose for RNA and deoxyribose for DNA (Figure 1). There are only four heterocyclic bases for most DNA or RNA: adenine, cytosine, guanine, and thymine (uracil for RNA). A ß–glycosyl linkage exists between the sugar and one of the four bases to form a nucleoside (Figure 2). The phosphate group is linked to either 3' or 5'-hydroxyl group of the sugar to form the nucleotide (Figure 3). This unit, the nucleotide, is the basic building block of the DNA and RNA which are polynucleotides.

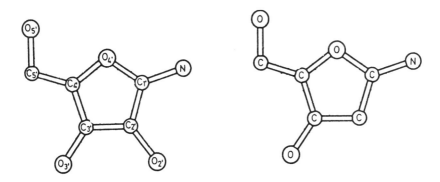

FIG. 1. The structures and numbering system of ribose (left) and 2'–deoxyribose (right). 0–4' is also numbered as 0–5 or 0–1'. Note also that the hydrogen atoms are not included.

83

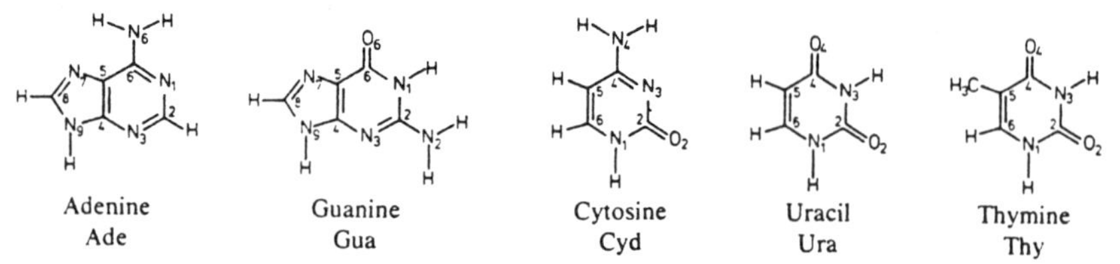

FIG. 2. The structures and numbering system of common nucleic acid bases.

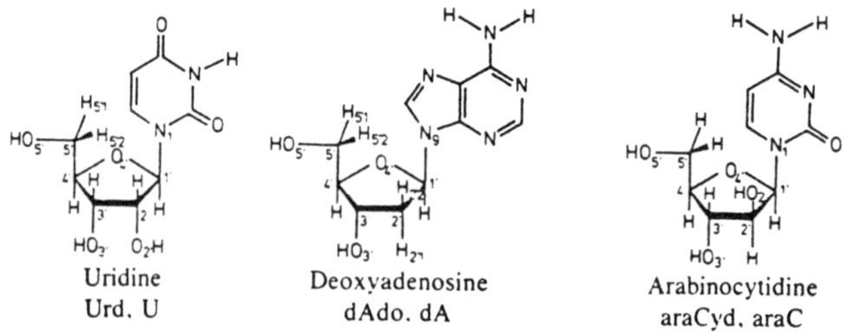

FIG. 3. The glycosyl linkage in the nucleoside. Please note that nucleic acid involves only one diastereoisomer of furanose.

BASES, NUCLEOSIDE AND NUCLEOTIDE

One way to understand how nucleic acid expresses its biological functions, is to understand its structure. For the studies of the structure of the block units of nucleic acid, such as the bases, nucleosides and nucleotides, the most powerful method is x–ray crystallography. This was pioneered by Furberg who published the crystal structure of cytidine in 1951 (21) (Figure 4). About two decades later, Voet and Rich (52) summarized more than one hundred structures of various purines and pyrimidines. Thus, the bond angles and bond lengths of these compounds were determined with 3° and 0.05 Å accuracy, respectively (Figure 5).

THE CONFORMATION OF NUCLEIC ACIDS

In general, the phosphate links the nucleosides between the 3' and 5' positions to form a nucleotidyl chain (Figure 7). Due to the similarity of the sugar–phosphate backbone of each nucleotidyl unit, the nomenclature of nucleic acid is usually dominated by the composition or the sequences of bases. For example, the segment of nucleic acid chain in Figure 7 is called r–A–G–U–C. The r is the symbol for ribonucleic acid and d is the designation for deoxyribonucleic acid and the sign (–) is for sugar–phosphate backbone. The sequence or the direction of the chain is from the free 5'–OH end toward the free 3'–OH end (Figure 7).

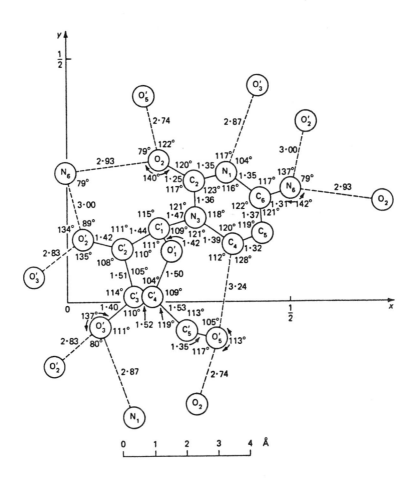

FIG. 4. The structure of cytidine by x-ray diffraction analysis. Bond lengths are given in angstroms. Hydrogen bond distances are indicated by broken lines. Note the C-4 is now numbered as C-6 in current nomenclature. From (21).

The 5'-3' phosphodiester linkage of the nucleic acid backbone is repeatable in every nucleotide, and it is convenient to designate the backbone structure between two adjacent phosphorus atoms as a vector for conformation and structure study. As shown in Figure 8, this vector consists of six free rotable single bonds and a five-membered ring structure (Table I). The different conformations of nucleic acid are the result of the myriad combinations of those rotatable bonds in the vector.

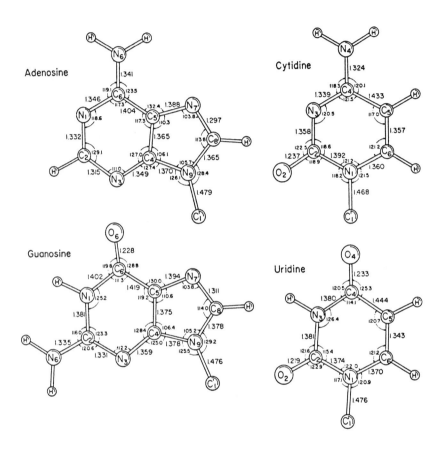

FIG. 5. Bond lengths (Å) and bond angles (°) of four bases from x–ray diffraction study. No ring atom is located more than 0.1 Å away from the calculated plane (by least–square method) for all ring atoms of purine and pyrimidine bases. For the structure of the sugar ring, three or four atoms of the five–membered ring will be coplanar, with the remaining one or two atoms displaced from the plane. In general, in DNA or RNA, either C–2' or C–3' atom is displaced by 0.5–0.6 Å from the plane. The out–of–plane atom(s) may be located either on the same side or the opposite side of the C–5' atom, designated as the <u>endo</u> or <u>exo</u> conformation, respectively (Figure 6) (24).

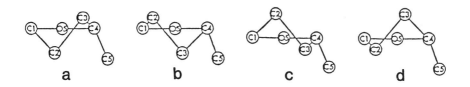

FIG. 6. Projections parallel to the C–1' to 0–1' to C–4' plane to show the four discrete modes of sugar ring puckering (deoxy–)ribose, C–2' and C–3' are either ≃ 0.5 or ≃ 0.1 Å distant from the reference plane. (a) C–2'–<u>endo</u>; (b) C–3'–<u>endo</u>; (c) C–2'–<u>exo</u>; (d) C–3'–<u>exo</u>. The definitions of <u>endo</u> and <u>exo</u> are described in the text.

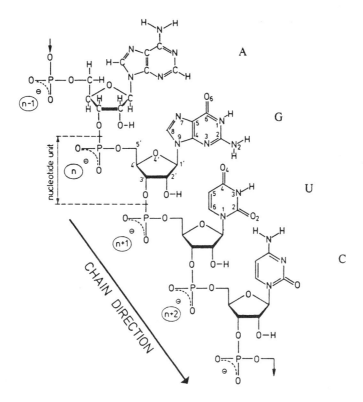

FIG. 7. Fragment of ribonucleic acid (RNA) with sequence adenosine (A), guanosine (G), uridine (U), cytidine (C) linked by 3',5'–phosphodiester bonds. Chain direction is from 5'–3'–end as shown by arrow. In short notation, this fragment would be r–pA–G–U–Cp.

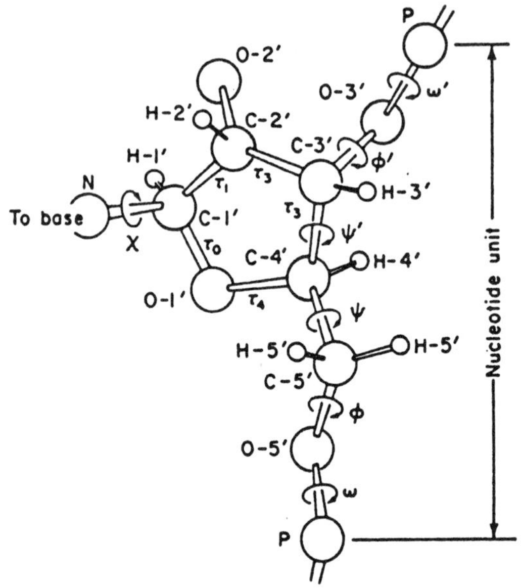

FIG. 8. The chemical bonds along the phosphodiester linkage of the nucleic acid backbone. See Table I for values of various torsion angles. From (48).

TABLE I. Definition of torsion angles in nucleotides (From 48)[a]

Torsion angle	Atoms involved
α	$(n-1)O_3'-P-O_5'-C_5'$
β	$P-O_5'-C_5'-C_4'$
γ	$O_5'-C_5'-C_4'-C_3'$
δ	$C_5'-C_4-C_3'-O_3'$
ε	$C_4'-C_3'-O_3'-P$
ζ	$C_3'-O_3'-P-O_5'(n+1)$
χ	$O_4'-C_1'-N_1-C_2$ (pyrimidines)
	$O_4'-C_1'-N_9-C_4$ (purines)
ν_0	$C_4'-O_4'-C_1'-C_2'$
ν_1	$O_4'-C_1'-C_2'-C_3'$
ν_2	$C_1'-C_2'-C_3'-C_4'$
ν_3	$C_2'-C_3'-C_4'-O_4'$
ν_4	$C_3'-C_4'-O_4'-C_1'$

[a] Atoms designated (n–1) and (n+1) belong to adjacent units.

A. The Rotation of the Glycosyl Linkage — The Syn and Anti Conformations

As described previously, the bases of the purine and pyrimidine are rigid planes, and the furanose ring only allows small ripples. In addition, these two planes are nearly perpendicular to each other in a nucleoside (Figure 9). Thus, the conformational state of the nucleoside is defined principally by the rotation of these two relatively rigid planes connected by C-1' to N-9 bond, in a purine nucleoside or to N-1 bond in a pyrimidine nucleoside, the glycosyl linkage. The sugar–base torsion angle, ϕCN, was first defined by Donohue and Trueblood as: "the angle formed by the trace of the plane of the base with the projection of the C-1' to O-1' bond of the furanose ring when viewed along the C-1' to N bond. This angle will be taken as zero when the furanose–ring oxygen atom is antiplanar to C-2 of the pyrimidine or purine ring, and positive angles will be taken as those measured in a clockwise direction when viewing from C-1' to N". (19). A graphic definition of the angle is shown in Figure 10. Donohue and Trueblood further concluded that there are two ranges of the torsion angle for the nucleosides: ca. -30°C for the anti and ca. +150° for the syn conformation. However, this torsion angle has been re-defined by Sundaralingam (45), Arnott (4), Sasisekharan and Lakshminarayanan (37) in their comprehensive works on the stereochemistry of nucleic acids based on the x-ray diffraction results as χ. The definiton of χ is demonstrated in Figure 11. In general, $\chi = \phi CN - 90°$.

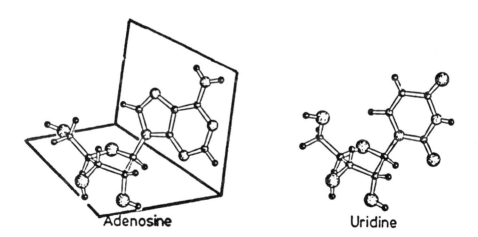

FIG. 9. The configuration of base and pentose planes.

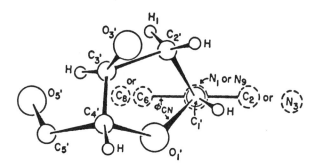

FIG. 10. Schematic illustration of the torsion angle in a pyrimidine or purine nucleoside. The plane of the base is viewed end–on with the glycosyl bond between C–1' and N–1 (or N–9) of the base perpendicular to the paper. The torsion angle (ϕCN) is the dihedral angle between the plane of the base and the plane formed by the C–1' to O–1' bond of the furanose ring and the C–1' to N–1 bond. The angle is zero when O–1' lies directly in front of C–6 (or C–8 for a purine), and positive angles are measured when C–1' to O–1' is rotated in a clockwise direction when viewing from C–1' to N.

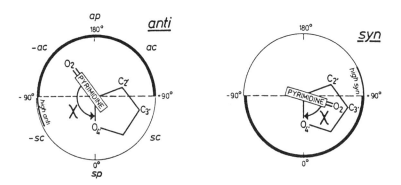

FIG. 11. Definition of <u>anti</u> and <u>syn</u> conformational ranges shown for pyrimidine nucleoside, χ is defined as torsion angle $O_4'-C_1'-N_1-C_2$. The pyrimidine base is toward the viewer; the base is rotated relative to the sugar. From (37).

B. The Sugar Puckering: The Pseudo Rotation Cycle

As mentioned previously, usually the sugar ring has four atoms in a plane and the fifth atom and out by 0.5 Å. This conformation is called the envelope form (E). Another conformation is the twist form (T) with two adjacent atoms displaced on opposite sides of a plane formed by the other three atoms (3). Since the absolute values of the displacement of T form is less than that of the E form, the sugar ring is still close to a plane (25) (Figure 12). It should be noted that because the transition between E and T forms is facile, usually the atoms defining the four–atom planes are not perfectly coplanar, and displacements from a three–atom plane are rarely symmetrical. Thus, the largest deviation from planarity is called major puckering; the lesser deviation is called minor puckering. The pseudo–rotation cycle of furanose ring in nucleoside can be reconstructed (25).

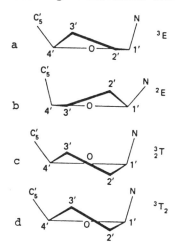

FIG. 12. Definition of sugar puckering modes. (a) Envelope $C_{3'}$–endo, ^3E. (b) Envelope $C_{2'}$–endo, ^2E. (c) Symmetrical twist or half–chair $C_{2'}$–exo-$C_{3'}$–endo, ^3_2T. (d) Unsymmetrical twist with major $C_{3'}$–endo and minor $C_{2'}$–exo pucker, $^3T_2$. Also, please refer to Figure 6.

C. C–4'–C–5' Bond

The rotation of the exocyclic C–4'–C–5' bond is very important to the conformation of the nucleic acid because it displaces the O–5' position relative to the furanose ring. Three possible rotation isomers are shown in Figure 13 (8).

D. The Phosphodiester Linkage

The phosphate group displays a tetrahedral configuration with P–O bond lengths varying from 1.5 Å for P–O (ion) to 1.6 Å for P–O (ester). The O–P–O angle is in a range of 105° to 120° (2). Figure 14 demonstrates the three possible conformations of C–3'–O–P–O–C–5' phosphodiester linkage.

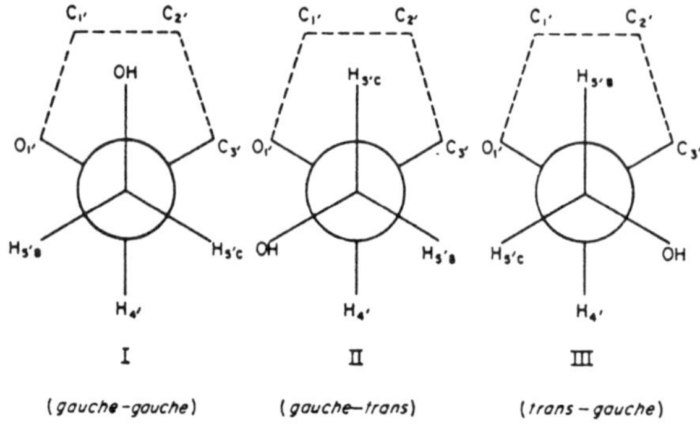

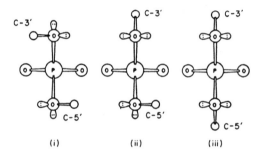

FIG. 13. Three conformers along C–4'–C–5' bond.

FIG. 14. The phosphodiester conformation. The electrostatic repulsion of the lone–pair electrons of the two oxygen atoms causes the <u>gauche–gauche</u> conformation (i), or <u>gauche–anti</u> conformation (ii) to be preferred conformation. The <u>anti–anti</u> conformation (iii) is not preferred due to this repulsion effect even though this extended conformation has less steric hindrance. From (45).

E. Helical Structure

The most unique feature of nucleic acid is the formation of double stranded helix which consists of two polynucleotide chains connected through complementary base pairing (Figure 15) (17, 19). The base pairs propel themselves to form helical turns (Figure 16). The base pairs are similar in shape with identical C–1' to C–1' distance between the two strands. The dyad axis connects C–6 of pyrimidine to C–8 of purine. Base–pairs are usually not centered on the helix axis but rather are displaced by a distance (D) (Figure 16). Owing to the branching off of the two glycosyl bonds from one side of the base–pairs, and owing to the displacement of the base–pairs by a distance D from the helix axis, the outer envelope of the double helix is not cylindrically smooth but can display two grooves of different width and depth (Figure 16).

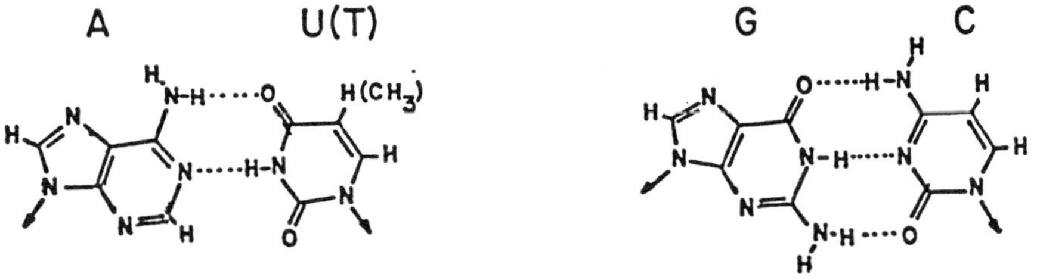

A U(T) G C

FIG. 15. A schematic diagram showing the standard Watson–Crick base pairs.

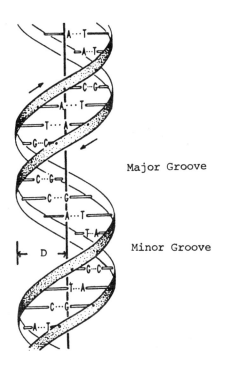

Major Groove

Minor Groove

D

FIG. 16. Schematic drawing of the DNA double helix. The sugar–phosphate backbones run at the periphery of the helix in anti–parallel orientation. Base-pairs (A–T and G–C) drawn symbolically as bars between chains are stacked along the center of the helix.

WHY NUCLEAR MAGNETIC RESONANCE SPECTROSCOPY IS USEFUL TO STUDY NUCLEIC ACID

X–ray crystallography, potential energy calculation, and spectroscopy are basic methods to elucidate the structure of nucleic acid. Potential energy calculations allow us to derive a general picture of the flexibility of a molecule. They are frequently used in structure refinement of macromolecules. X–ray crystal structure analyses generate unambiguous results, but are limited in the ordered, solid state. The general spectroscopic method employed on the studies of nucleic acids are UV and IR absorption, circular dichroism, laser Raman, fluorescence, etc.

(for review 9,11,42,47,48), as well as nuclear magnetic resonance spectroscopy (NMR). Among these methods, NMR yields the most detailed information at atomic level and also at the ground state (not the excited state) through the investigation of the nuclei having magnetic spins, such as ^{1}H, ^{13}C, ^{15}N, and ^{31}P. In addition, NMR studies are conducted in aqueous solution and will shed light on dynamic properties. In order to effectively utilize this approach, we must be familiar with the type of information gained by NMR:

A. Chemical Shifts (δ, in ppm)

This parameter gives the intrinsic, chemical properties of the nucleus, as well as the magnetic field of the immediate nuclear environment. The external fields exerted by the nearby atoms or groups of atoms, as detected by their chemical shifts, provide the most valuable information about the conformation and through–space interaction of biopolymers in solution.

B. Coupling Constants (J, in Hz)

This parameter reveals the interactions of neighboring magnetic dipoles. It can provide the valence and spatial relationship between the atom of interest and nearby atoms. At present, coupling constant is most useful for the evaluation of the dihedral angles determined by a three–bond coupling constant, ^{3}J, through the application of Karplus equation (34). The relationship of torsion angle and dihedral angle is illustrated in Figure 17.

C. Intensities of the Resonance Lines

This parameter provides information about the number of the equivalent nuclei on a function group. In order to make the result valid, an internal standard is necessary.

D. Relaxation Times

There are two kinds of relaxation times: spin–lattice relaxation time, or T_1, which denotes the relaxation rate of the absorbed energy dissipation from the (hot) spin–system to the lattice; and spin–spin relaxation time, or T_2, which denotes the relaxation rate through the spin redistribution. Thus, these two parameters indicate the kinetics of the interaction between the nearby spins and their environments.

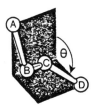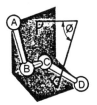

FIG. 17. Definition of torsion (ϕ) and dihedral (θ) angles; $\phi + \theta = 180°$.

E. Nuclear Overhauser Effect (NOE)

The definition of NOE is quite simple: a variation in the signal intensity of spin 1, produced when the resonances of spin 2, which interacts with 1 through relaxation, are saturated by means of a complementary radio frequency (RF). Thus, we can take advantage to obtain the spatial relationship of spins close to each other through space (41).

THE GENERAL APPROACHES OF ^{1}H NMR STUDIES OF NUCLEIC ACIDS

A. Resonance Signals Assignment

To reveal the identity of resonance signal is essential for further study and this can be approached by many ways.

(a) By chemical shift values: There are four regions for nucleic acid. The C–2' protons of deoxyribofuranose and the methyl group of T appear in the region of 1 to 2.5 ppm when DSS (2,2–dimethyl–2–silapentane–5–sulfonate) was used as an internal standard. C–2' (in RNA), C–3', –4' and –5' protons resonate in an area of 3 to 5.5 ppm. C–1' and C–5 of pyrimidine bases are in 5.5 to 6.5 ppm and the C–8 proton of purine base C–2 proton of adenine and C–6 proton of pyrimidine base resonate in a region of 7 to 8.5 ppm. These are the non–labile protons so they can be detected even in D_2O (in which the labile or exchangeable protons will be replaced by the deuterium) as shown in Figure 18. The important labile proton is the NH protons. NH protons resonate in 9–11 ppm when they are not hydrogen bonded, shift to 12–15 ppm if they involve hydrogen bonding. This observation serves as a remarkable indicator for the existence of double stranded helix and will be discussed later. The ^{1}H NMR spectrum will become more complex for the longer nucleic acid chain, since the protons in the same category from each nucleoside unit will appear in the same region. Thus, these signals will pile on top of each other, causing difficulties in resolution.

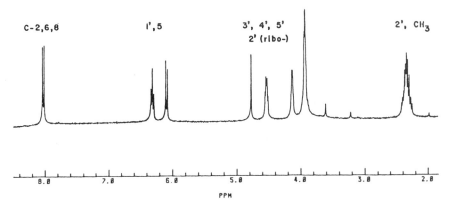

FIG. 18. ^{1}H NMR spectrum of 5'–d–CMP in D_2O. The designation of chemical shift regions are on the top of peaks.

(b) <u>By resonating pattern</u>. Since each chemical group may have a different magnetic environment, so their NMR signal patterns may also be different. C–2, C–8 of purine base are singlets; C–5 and C–6 of cytosine and uracil, C–6 and methyl group of thymine are also coupled, except the latter pair has a very small coupling constant. The furanose ring protons are multiplets with different characteristics. For example, the pattern of C–5' protons are different if a phosphate group is linked to the OH group (30).

(c) <u>By isotope substitution</u>. Usually the deuterium is used for substitution of hydrogen. Since deuterium will not be detected by ^{1}H NMR, the identity of hydrogen which has been substituted by deuterium, can be readily revealed by comparison between the spectra of the original compound and the specifically deuterium substituted compound. The three purine ring proton resonances were assigned by this classical method in the beginning of the NMR study of nucleic acid (44). This method is commonly used to assign the C–8 proton of adenosine and guanosine due to its acidic property of the proton, allowing this proton to exchange with D_2O at high temperature (49). This method is useful especially for the assignment of proton resonances originating from the same unit but at different sequence location of an oligonucleotide.

(d) <u>By spin–lattice relaxation time T_1</u>. This is an effective procedure to distinguish C–2 and C–8 proton of purine type base. The T_1 value of C–2 proton signal is much longer than that of C–8 proton, since this proton is close to the C–5'–phosophate group in an <u>anti</u> conformation (50).

(e) <u>By comparison with various smaller fragments</u>. This is a powerful method for assignment of ^{1}H resonances in oligonucleotides up to ten nucleotidyl units, when the shorter fragments are available either as by–products, or as the building blocks of the longer oligomer. In Figure 19, we demonstrate the usage of this method to unambiguously assign the ^{1}H resonances from the two oligomers, r–A–A–G–C–U–U and d–C–C–A–A–G–C–T–T–G–G. The assignment of ^{1}H resonances of r–A–A was made in our laboratory previously (36) and has been confirmed by the deuterium substitution method (35). Thus, the assignments of ^{1}H resonances of r–A–A–G, r–A–A–G–C, r–A–A–G–C–U, and r–A–A–G–C–U–U can be done sequentially and incrementally by comparison of the longer fragments with the shorter fragments. Similarly, the proton resonances of d–C–C–A–A–G–C–T–T–G–G have been identified in the same procedure. It would be possible but tedious to compare all the fragments incrementally from two to nine nucleotidyl units in length. Thus, the ^{1}H resonances of this decamer is assigned with the aid of two pentamers (two halves of the decamer). The ^{1}H resonances of these two pentamers were identified by the same approach earlier.

(f) <u>By scalar coupling connectivity</u>. Scalar coupling measurement is limited to three covalent bonds in distance since the coupling constant of four or more bond distances is usually very small. Thus, the protons in one nucleotidyl unit have no scalar coupling to protons of its neighbor unit carbon. This method is useful to identify the relationship between C–5 and C–6 protons of cytosine but more importantly, for furanose ring protons

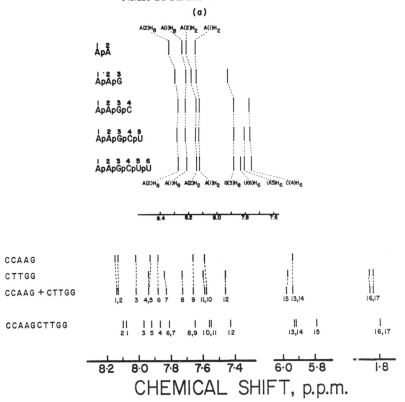

CHEMICAL SHIFT, p.p.m.

FIG. 19. The incremental assignment scheme for all the base resonances of r-A-A-G-C-U-U (left) and d-C-C-A-A-G-C-T-T-G-G (right). The numbering system of peaks is the following. $1 = A^4-H_8$; $3 = A^4-H_2$; $5 = G^{10}-H_8$; $6 = G^5-H_8$; $7 = G^9-H_8$; $8 = C^6-H_6$; $9 = C^1-H_6$; $10 = C^2-H_6$; $11 = T^7-H_6$; $12 = T^8-H_6$; $13 = C^1-H_5$; $14 = C^2-H_5$; $15 = C^6-H_5$; $16 = T^7-CH_3$; $17 = T^8-CH_3$, where $d-C^1-C^2-A^3-A^4-G^5-G^5-C^6-T^7-T^8-G^9-G^{10}$. From (10, 20).

which couple to each other when connected through the adjacent carbons. Thus, either double resonance technique and/or two–dimensional NMR spectroscopy can be employed to reveal the connectivity of these ^{1}H resonances. A scalar coupling connectivity correlated 2D NMR (termed COSY) (7) spectrum of 5'-d-CMP is shown as a contour plot in Figure 20. As presented in this plot, the spectrum is being viewed down from the top, thus every signal becomes a spot. The regular 1D NMR spectrum in Figure 20 is displayed on the diagonal line from lower left corner to upper right corner (compare to Figure 18). Off diagonal points will show up for those resonances coupled together. Thus, one can simply 'walk' through the assignment of all furanose protons (as illustrated by the arrows). The spectrum of oligomer will be more complicated but the same approach can be applied, all the connected sugar proton identities can be ascertained starting with one known assignment (usually C-1' proton, see next section).

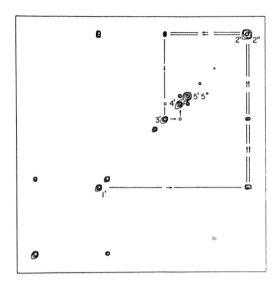

FIG. 20. 2D COSY of 5'–d–CMP.

(g) <u>By nuclear Overhauser effect (NOE)</u>. According to the x–ray crystallography studies, in the generalized B conformation, the C–8 (or C–6) proton of the nth nucleotidyl unit of an oligonucleotide is close to its own C–2'H' and to C–2'H" of the furanose of the (n–1)th nucleotidyl unit (see Figure 7). Figure 21 demonstrates this relationship via a molecule of d–C–G–C–G–C–G (shown by arrows). Thus, the spatial proximity of (n–1)H2"↔(n)H8 (or H6)↔(n)H2'↔(n)H2"↔(n+1)H8 (or H6) can be observed through the NOE experiment (20). In addition the C–8 (or C–6) proton is also close to its own C–1' proton. Thus, the 'walk' through assignment technique can be carried out from one nucleotidyl unit to the next unit in an oligonucleotide chain. Similar to scalar coupling relationship, the NOE can be detected either by double resonance technique or by two–dimensional NOE spectroscopy (2D NOESY) (39).

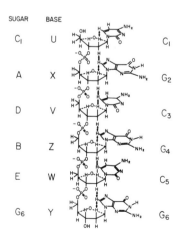

FIG. 21. The spatial relationship of the protons in d–G–G–C–G–C–G, with the arrows connect the scheme of assignment of proton resonances from one end to the other end by NOE. From (20).

In addition, the 2D NOESY can be used to assign the NH–N hydrogen bonded proton resonance in an oligomer in H_2O solution. This is because the two adjacent base pairs are close enough to exert the NOE to each others NH–N resonance. Thus, the end base–pair which has only one neighbor will have a different NOE pattern than that of the internal base–pairs. For this reason, one can again 'walk' the assignment from one end to the other end or to the middle of the helix which has a self–complementary sequence. Furthermore, the N_3–H of T base is also close to C–2 proton of A base in A–T base–pair (Figure 22). Thus, one can recognize which NH–N is from A–T base pair by examining the NOE on C2 proton.

Thus, one can recognize which NH–N is from A–T base pair by examining the NOE on C2 proton. Hence, by a combination of above discussed methods, the ^1H NMR resonances of an oligonucleotide can usually be assigned.

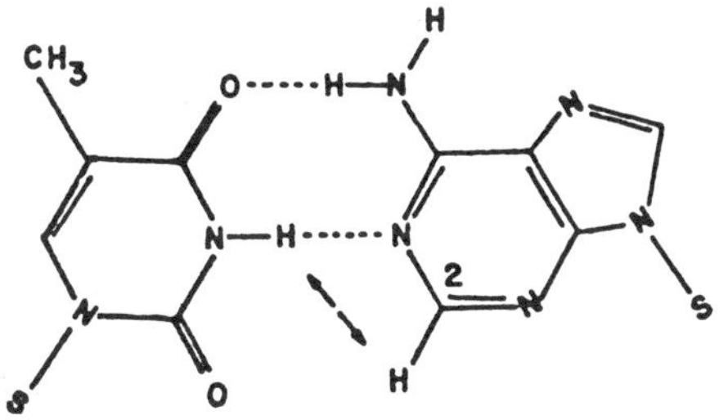

FIG. 22. Watson–Crick hydrogen–binding scheme of an adenine–thymine base pair. In this figure the short distance (2.84 Å) between the N_3–H of T to the C_2–H of A indicated by an arrow. S represents the position of the C_1' atom of the deoxyfuranose residue. From (31).

B. The Study of Chemical Shift —
The Conformation of Base–Base Stacking

Once the assignment of the ^1H resonances is done, the structure and conformation of nucleic acid can be studied by all the NMR parameters described above. Figures 23 and 24 showed the chemical shift profiles of non–exchangeable proton resonances of r–A–A–G–C–U–U and d–C–C–A–A–G–C–T–T–G–G (10,29). Thus, the change of chemical shift of each base proton signal in an oligomer can be calculated with respect to that from the corresponding monomer. Furthermore, the spatial magnetic field effects on chemical shift can be calculated from the general A'–, A–, and B–DNA conformation defined by x–ray diffraction data (5,6) and from the ring current magnetic anisotropy (22,31). The conclusions based on comparison between the observed and calculated chemical shift differences showed that r–A–A–G–C–U–U and d–C–C–A–A–G–C–T–T–G–G can be rationalized to be in A'– and B–DNA conformation, respectively (10,29). Furthermore, a similar conclusion can be drawn based on same studies on the chemical shifts of NH–N proton resonances observed in H_2O solution (26,29).

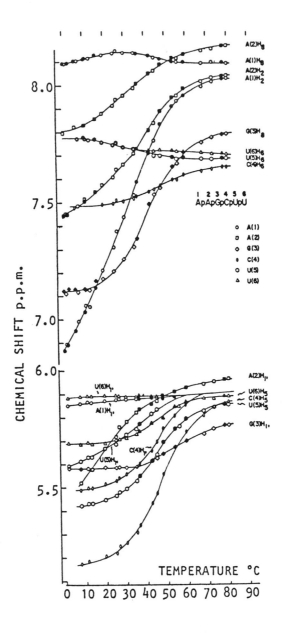

FIG. 23. The plot of the chemical shifts of base and $H_{1'}$ protons of r–A–A–G–C–U–U in D_2O (10 mM in strand concentration, 0.01 M sodium phosphate buffer, pD = 7.0, 0.07 M Na^+) versus temperature. All chemical shifts are expressed in reference to DSS. The solid symbols represent the data from the 100 MHz spectrometer and the open symbols represent the data from the 220 MHz spectrometer. From (10).

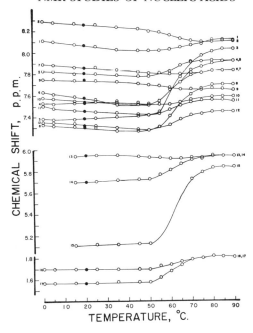

FIG. 24. Profiles of the chemical shift data of non–exchangeable base proton resonances of d–C–C–A–A–G–C–T–T–G–G vs. temperature. The peak numbering system is the same as in Figure 19. The open circles represent data which were obtained at 360 MHz and closed circles the data obtained at 600 MHz. From (29).

The chemical shift parameter is also useful for conformation determination of more complicated nucleic acid, such as transfer RNA (tRNA). We have studied the methyl and methylene proton resonances of tRNA^{phe} (Figure 25) from yeast (32). The chemical shift versus temperature profile of methyl and methylene group signals is shown in Figure 26.

The results in this comparison can be classified into four categories. The first category contains seven resonances, $m_2^2G_{26}$ (average position of two methyl groups) Cm_{32}, Gm_{34}, Y_{37} (all 4 methyl resonances) and m^5C_{40}. The observed and the calculated chemical shift changes ($\Delta\delta$) of these seven resonances are in agreement with each other within 0.1 ppm. Since these four modified residues are either in anticodon loops or in the anticodon stem, the results suggest no difference in the conformations of anticodon stem and the anticodon loop of this tRNA in aqueous solution versus that in the crystalline state (43) can be found by this approach.

The second category contains $m_2^2G_{10}$, $D_{16,17}(C_5)$, $D_{16,17}(C_6)$ and m^5C_{49}. The observed $\Delta\delta$ of these resonances in this category are much higher (more than 0.1 ppm) than the calculated $\Delta\delta$, indicating these protons are more shielded than the predicted values based on crystal structure and ring–current effects. Whiel there exists some doubt about the assignment of $D_{16,17}(C_6)$ resonance in the native tRNA spectrum, this conclusion is most likely correct, since it is supported by the results on $D_{16,17}(C_5)$.

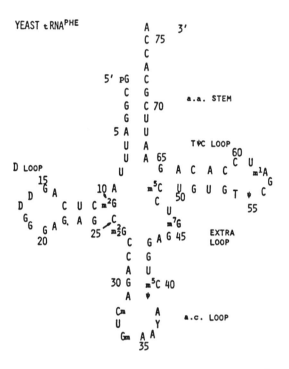

FIG. 25. The cloverleaf structure of Baker's yeast tRNAphe.

The third category contains m⁷G₄₆ and m¹A₅₈. The observed Δδ of these two resonances are much lower (0.15–0.20 ppm) than the calculated Δδ, indicating these protons are <u>less</u> shielded than the predicted values based on crystal structure and ring–current effects.

Finally, the fourth category contains a T residue. The methyl resonance from T has only one predicted ring–current effect value but two Δδ values are observed (32). However, both experimental values are not in good agreement with the predicted value (interestingly, one was too high and the other too low).

In summary, the comparison indicates that no differences between observed and calculated Δδ values from resonances in the anticodon stem and loop can be found, but differences in the TψC stem/loop and D stem/loop have been uncovered. The nature of the results, with both agreement and disagreement involving values that are too high or too low, suggests that the difference may indeed be due to the difference in conformation.

A similar approach is being used for the hydrogen–bonded NH–N resonances of yeast tRNAphe (33). The difference in this case is that the resonances have not been assigned with certainty.

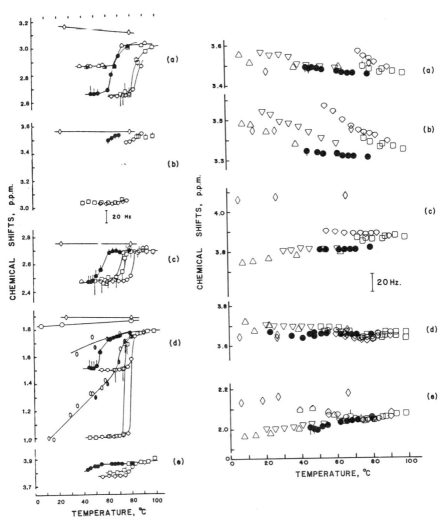

FIG. 26. Left: The chemical-shift data of the methyl proton resonances from (a) m$_2^2$G, (b) D', (c) D, (d) T, and (e) m^{1}A in the monomer, the intact tRNA^{phe}, and its fragments vs. temperature. The explanation of the symbols used is as follows: (◇) the monomer; (○) fragment 54–58; (□) fragment 1–45 in 0.01 M MgCl$_2$; (◐) fragment 47–76 in 0.01 M MgCl$_2$; (●) yeast tRNA^{phe}; (□) yeast tRNA^{phe} in 0.01 M MgCl$_2$.

Right: The chemical-shift data of the methyl proton resonances from (a) Cm, (b) Gm, (c) Y", (d) Y', and (e) Y, of the monomer, intact tRNA^{phe} and fragment 31–42 and fragment 1–45 vs. temperatures, where Δ represents fragment 31–42 and ▽ represents the fragment 31–41 in 0.1 M NaCl and 0.1 M MgCl$_2$. From (32).

Figure 27 shows the 360 MHz spectrum of the ^{1}H NMR resonances of the hydrogen–bonded NH from yeast tRNA^{phe} sample at 23°C. Under this condition, the spectrum is essentially insensitive to temperature variation with ± 10°C and can be considered as a reliable representation of the hydrogen–bonded NH resonances of yeast tRNA^{phe} in native conformation. This spectrum has a good signal–to–noise ratio, and contains 15 well–resolved peaks plus a shoulder (k') in the region of 11 to 15 ppm for DSS.

The interatomic/intermolecular magnetic field experienced by the NH–N resonances in yeast tRNA^{phe} was then calculated based on the ring current effect, as evaluated from the coordinates derived from the x–ray diffraction data (33). This result was plotted by the PDP–10 computer as shown in Figure 27. The adjustments needed to transform the computed spectrum to the simulated experimental spectrum are shown between Figures 27 middle and bottom. This computed spectrum contains 23 resonances, six resonances less than the total recommneded by the three dimensional structure of tRNA determined by x–ray diffraction.

In conclusion, despite some uncertainties in the theoretical treatment, this quantitative comparison between the simulated experimental spectrum and the calculated spectrum based on the atomic coordinates of the tRNA in crystal and on ring–current effects clearly indicates that the native conformation of yeast tRNA^{phe} in solution is fundamentally similar to that in the crystalline state. The minor difference is probably in the tertiary structure involving the folding of the TψC loop and stem to the D loop and stem. This conclusion is reinforced by the ^{1}H NMR studies on the methyl/methylene resonances of the minor bases reported above. In addition, some of the hydrogen–bonded base pairs existing in the tRNA in the crystalline state may not be detectable in solution.

C. The Studies by Coupling Constants–Sugar–Phosphate Backbone Conformation

The vicinal coupling constant (^{3}J) has been shown to be related to the dihedral angle of a A–X–Y–B spin system (Figure 17) (34). In the case of the couplings of H–C–C'–H' system in the furanose ring, the following relationship was found by Lemieux, et al. (38).

$$^3J = Jo \cos^2\phi - 0.28$$

where ^{3}J is the vicinal coupling constant, ϕ is the dihedral angle between H–C–C' and the C–C'–H' planes in a fragment of H–C–C'–H' in the furanose (Figure 17). From the experimental results, Jo = 9.27 Hz for ϕ below 90° and Jo = 10.36 Hz for ϕ above 90° were calibrated. In general, the furanose ring pucker falls into one of two conformers (i.e. C–2' endo for B–DNA and C–3' endo for A–DNA) for which the J of C–1' and C–2' protons are different. The ^{3}J(1'–2') can be calculated as 0.4 Hz and 8.6 Hz for C–3' and C–2' endo, respectively. Thus, conformation of furanose ring

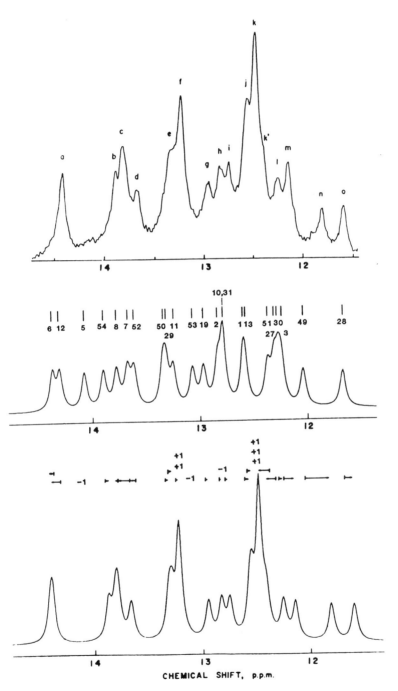

FIG. 27.   See legend on next page.

FIG. 27. Top: A 360 MHz spectrum of the yeast tRNA^{phe} at the 11.5–14.5 ppm region from DSS showing the hydrogen–bonded NH resonances at 23°C. The sample contained 25 mg/ml of tRNA^{phe}, dissolved in 0.01 M MgCl$_2$, 0.15 M NaCl, 0.002 M EDTA and 0.01 M potassium phosphate buffer, pH 7.0.

Middle: The computed spectrum of NH–N hydrogen–bonded proton resonances. The number of these NH resonances represent the following base pairs: 6:U$_6$A$_{67}$, 12:U$_{12}$A$_{23}$, 5:A$_5$U$_{68}$, 54:T$_{54}$m^{1}A$_{58}$, 7:U$_7$A$_{66}$, 8:U$_8$A$_{14}$, 52:U$_{52}$A$_{62}$, 50:U$_{50}$A$_{64}$, 29:A$_{29}$U$_{41}$, 11:C$_{11}$G$_{24}$, 53:G$_{53}$C$_{61}$, 19:G$_{19}$C$_{56}$, 2:C$_2$G$_{71}$, 10:m^{2}G$_{10}$C$_{25}$, 31:A$_{31}$ $_{39}$, 1:G$_1$G$_{72}$, 13:C$_{13}$G$_{22}$, 51:G$_{51}$C$_{63}$, 27:C$_{27}$G$_{43}$, 30:G$_{30}$m^{5}C$_{40}$, 3:G$_3$C$_{70}$, 49:m^{5}C$_{49}$C$_{65}$, and 28:C$_{28}$G$_{42}$. Every computed peak has an equal linewidth at half–height; 36 Hz in 360 MHz scale.

Bottom: A simulated spectrum. Every peak has a 36 Hz linewidth at half–height in 360 MHz scale. The symbols represent the adjustments needed to transform the computed spectrum to the simulated spectrum: (–) represents removal of resonance peaks, (+) represents addition of resonance peaks, and → or ← represent moving the chemical shifts to high or low field, respectively.

can be determined by the ^{3}J(1'–2') value. Figure 28 shows the J(1'–2') in Hz of r–A–A–G–C–U–U (10) versus temperature (as well as a function of salt concentration). The ^{3}J values are near 5 Hz at high temperature which indicates an equilibrium of C–2' and C–3' endo conformation existing in a single stranded state. However, the ^{3}J values were decreasing when temperature became lower. This result indicates that the conformation of furanose ring in r–A–A–G–C–U–U assumes a C–3' endo conformation in the helical state as expected in the A form. In contrast, the ^{3}J(1'–2') of d–C–C–A–A–G–C–T–T–G–G did not decrease as temperature was lowered (29). This data indicates that the sugar conformation of d–C–C–A–A–G–C–T–T–G–G is in C–2' endo conformation, as expected in the B–DNA conformation. These conclusions are in congruence with those obtained by chemical shift studies.

The other torsion angles in Figure 8 can also be detected by ^{3}J values:

Torsion angle	Coupling constants
χ	^{13}C–^{1}H
ψ	^{1}H–^{1}H
φ'	^{1}H–^{31}P
φ	^{1}H–^{31}P

only ω and ω' cannot be determined directly by NMR technique.

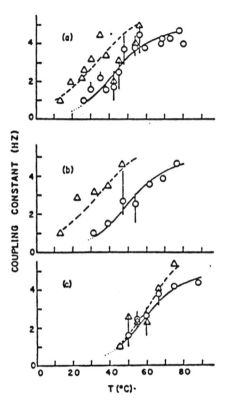

FIG. 28. The H'_1–H_2, coupling constants, $J_{1'-2'}$, for the six ribose H_1, resonances of r–A–A–G–C–U–U as a function of temperature and counterion concentration: (a) 0.07 M Na$^+$, (b) 0.17 M Na$^+$, (c) 1.07 M Na$^+$. The $J_{1'-2'}$ values for the tentatively identified U(6)H_1, signal (– – –) were plotted separately from the average of the other 5 resonances (——). The vertical bars indicate the range of values observed for these five signals and the lowest temperature point indicates the temperature at which all the resonances become singlets with $J_{1'-2'} < 1.5$ Hz. From (10).

The 500 MHz ^{1}H NMR studies of d–C–G–C–G and d–C–G–C–G–C–G in helical state provided a detailed result on the application of coupling constants (12). All coupling constants (listed in Table II) were obtained by computer simulation method (for example, the results of d–C–G–C–G–C–G are shown in Figure 29). Thus the percentage of C–2' <u>endo</u> conformers, the conformers along C–4'–C–5' bond, C–5'–O(P), and C–3'–O(P) bonds can be calculated based on the information in Table II, and the results are collected in Table III (12). The conformation of deoxyribofuranose of both d–C–G–C–G and d–C–G–C–G–C–G in helical form showed a clear preference to populate in C–2' <u>endo</u> form. The conformers around

TABLE II. Coupling Constants[a] of Sugar Protons of d–C–G–C–G and d–C–G–C–G–C–G[b] at Different Temperatures

Compounds	Temp. (°C)	1'2'	1'2"	2'2"	2'3'	2"3'	3'4'	4'5'	4'5"	5'5"	3'P	4'P	5'P	5"P
CGCG														
C^1	9	8.0	6.1	−14.0	6.7	2.6	3.0	3.1	4.0	−12.1	5.7	—	—	—
G^2		8.2	6.6	−14.0	6.4	2.7	2.0	2.4	2.0	−11.8	5.5	1.0	3.0	3.8
C^3		7.9	6.1	−14.0	6.8	2.5	2.7	3.0	3.0	−11.3	5.5	2.1	3.2	3.2
G^4		8.0	6.3	−14.0	6.0	2.6	2.5	3.1	3.1	−11.3	—	1.4	3.5	3.5
CGCGCG														
C^1	25	8.1	6.2	−14.0	6.2	2.9	3.2	3.6	5.0	−11.8	5.9	—	—	—
G^2		8.6	5.5	−14.3	6.3	1.7	2.8	~3.5	2.0	−11.6	5.8	2.0	3.8	4.0
C^3		8.5	5.6	−14.0	6.7	3.1	2.7	~2.8	~2.8	−11.3	5.8	2.0	~3.0	~3.0
G^4		8.5	5.5	−14.3	6.3	1.7	2.8	~3.5	2.0	−11.5	5.8	1.9	~3.8	4.2
C^5		8.3	6.4	−14.0	6.9	2.5	2.6	~2.8	~2.8	−11.3	5.8	2.0	~3.2	~3.2
G^6		8.0	6.0	−14.0	6.3	3.1	2.7	~3.0	~3.0	−11.3	—	2.0	~3.3	~3.3

[a] J_{H-H} or J_{H-P} (in Hz)

[b] In D_2O, pD 7.4, 0.02M $NaHPO_4$

[c] Under HDO

C–4'–C–5' and C–5'–O(P) bonds of these helical oligomers also showed clearly a preference for gauche–gauche and gauche'–gauche', respectively. The rotamer distributions about the C–3'–O(P) are in 195/285° range for both compounds. Thus, these two C–G alternate oligohelices in low salt condition are indeed in B–DNA form (12) in spite of the capability to form Z–form in high salt condition or in crystalline form (53).

Recently, the 2D–JRES (40) technique has been successfully applied to the study of nucleic acids (28). This technique may simplify the crowded sugar resonance region (Figure 29).

D. The Studies of the NH–N Hydrogen Bonded Proton Resonances

The detection of such resonances provides unambiguous evidence of the existence of base–pairing in the double stranded helix. This approach is applicable to not only the Watson–Crick type of base–pair (12,17,26,29), but also other types of base–pairs in tRNA (33), as well as the unusual G–A base pairs (27). Figure 30 shows the NH–N proton resonance of the self–association of d–C–C–A–A–G–A–T–T–G–G, a decamer. The outside

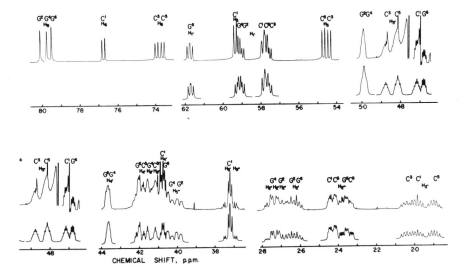

FIG. 29. 500–MHz ^{1}H–NMR spectrum of d–C–G–C–G–C–G at 25°C (600 scans), 350 O.D./ml, 0.02M phosphate buffer, pD 7.4, in D_2O. The line–shape simulation is shown at the bottom of the observed spectrum.

TABLE III. Conformation and Population Distribution of Conformers of the Sugar Backbone of d–C–G–C–G and d–C–G–C–G–C–G at Different Temperatures[a]

Compounds	Temp. (°C)	Helix (%)	^{2}E (%)	gg (%)	g'g' (%)	ϕ'
CGCG						
C^1	9	100	72	68	—	195°/285°
G^2			81	96	88	194°/286°
C^3			75	79	89	194°/286°
G^4			76	77	87	—
CGCGCG						
C^1	25	100	71	53	—	196°/284°
G^2			75	85	83	195°/285°
C^3			76	83	91	195°/285°
G^4			75	85	82	195°/285°
C^5			78	83	89	195°/285°
G^6			76	79	88	—

a ^{2}E = 100 – [$J_{3'4'}$/($J_{1'2'}$+$J_{3'4'}$)]x100; accurate to ±1–2%.
%gg = [(13.7–Σ)/9.7]x100; Σ = $J_{4'5'}$+$J_{4'5''}$; accurate to ±6–7%.
%g'g' = [(25–Σ')/20.8]x100; Σ' = $J_{5'p}$+$J_{5''p}$; accurate to ±6–7%.
$^3J_{HP}$ = 18.1cos$^2\theta_{HP}$ – 4.8cosθ_{HP}; ϕ' = 240° ± θ; accurate to ±3°.

four bases in each end are complementary, forcing the G and A to face each other in the middle of the helix. Clearly, there are five NH–N resonances in Figure 30; thus, one NH–N resonance may belong to G–A base pair. This prediction was verified by NOE and deuterium exchange technique (see Section a). In addition, the results also support that the conformation of both bases are in <u>anti</u> form (27).

Thus, the disappearance of these NH–N resonances reflects the dissociation of the base–pair. With this observation plus the measurement of linewidth at half-height, one can study the dynamics of helix formation (18). From reference 12, one may realize that the 'melting' of double stranded oligonucleotide helices is a 'zipper' type of process. This is because the NH–N resonance of C^1G^{10} disappeared first, followed by C^2G^9, sequentially toward the center of the helix (29). In order words, the dissociation of the helix is from end toward the middle, not necessarily following a 'none–or–all type' in this concentration and condition.

The linewidth of NH–N resonance can be used to estimate the lifetime of the base pair. For example, the lifetimes of external A–U, internal A–U and center G–C base pairs of r–A–A–G–C–U–U helix can be calculated as 4.1, 7.2 and 10.6 msec, respectively, at 1°C (26).

NMR STUDIES OF NUCLEI OTHER THAN HYDROGEN

A. ^{31}P NMR

^{31}P has a natural abundance of 100%, and the magnetic spin number of ^{31}P is one half; therefore, there is no quadrapole relaxation. More importantly, the phosphorus atom in the phosphate group is in a key position of sugar–phosphate backbone. It is well established that the magnetic shielding values of the phorphorus nucleus of the

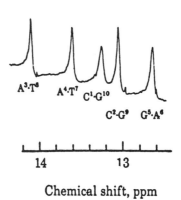

Chemical shift, ppm

FIG. 30. The NH–N hydrogen–bonded proton resonances of d–C^1–C^2–A^3–A^4–G^5–C^6–T^7–T^8–G^9–G^{10} duplex. From (27).

pentose–phosphate backbone of nucleic acids is very sensitive to the conformation of the phosphate group (24 and references therein). The variations observed have been attributed to the difference in the rotation angles about the P–O ester bonds and in the ester O–P–O bond angle. However, there is no correlation between these two factors (24). In addition, it was found that the conformation along the C–3'–O(P) and C–5'–O(P) bonds can also have a contribution as much as three ppm to the chemical shift of the phosphate phosphorus (23). This observation may add more complexities to the theoretical understanding of the chemical shift of phosphorus in nucleic acids.

Thus, the first step to study ^{31}P NMR in nucleic acid is to assign all the ^{31}P signals in the nucleic acid, starting with oligonucleotides. Fortunately, this mission becomes relatively easier after the thorough assignment of the ^{1}H NMR spectrum. This strategy is illustrated in Figure 31. The three phosphorus atoms in d–T–T–G–G scalar couples to C–3' and C–5' protons of two adjacent furanoses. Thus, the patterns of these ^{1}H resonances will be altered if their coupled phosphorus signal is irradiated (the shaded parts of Figure 31) (14). It is worthwhile to mention here that irradiation of ^{31}P needs a third frequency channel (13) of Bruker manufactured NMR spectrometer. Thus, the identities of three phosphorus resonances in d–T–T–G–G were revealed.

By taking advantage of this method, the phosphorus resonances of following oligonucleotides have been assigned with confidence:

d–C–C–A	d–T–G–G
d–C–C–A–A	d–T–T–G–G
d–C–C–A–A–G	d–C–T–T–G–G
d–C–C–A–A–G–A	
d–C–C–A–A–T	

In addition, the chemical shift values of all 16 dideoxyribose monophosphates have also been investigated. From the available data, we have deduced the following guidelines to assign the ^{31}P NMR signals in oligonucleotides (13).

(a) The 3'-end terminal phosphorus resonance in an oligomer tends to locate at a spectral position relatively close to its constitutive dimeric unit.

(b) On chain elongation (from 5'- toward 3'-end), the phosphorus resonance in the oligomer will be shifted upfield by 0.2–0.3 ppm, as compared to its constitutive dimeric unit.

(c) The relative positions of phosphorus resonances in an oligomer tend to remain in the same order as their constitutive dimeric units.

The validity of these guidelines can be tested, as shown in Figure 32. The assignment of the phosphorus resonances of d–C–C–A–A–T can be predicted by these guidelines and verified by the heterodecoupling techniques.

This important experimental observation provides a great incentive and impetus to current research aimed at providing the theoretical understanding of the chemical shift of phosphorus in oligonucleotides.

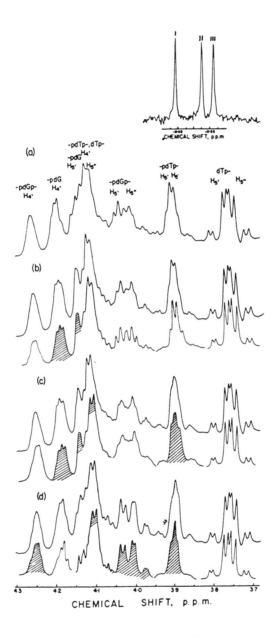

FIG. 31. (Insert) Totally proton–decoupled ^{31}P resonances of d–T–T–G–G.
(a) The C–4', C–5' proton resonances of d–T–T–G–G. (b) Same as (a)
except that peak 1 was irradiated; (c) Same as (a) except Peaks I and II
were irradiated. (d) Same as (a) except peaks II and III were irradiated.
From (14).

B. The Carbon Atom Is Ubiquitous in Biological Molecules

Unfortunately, the major isotope, carbon–12, has no magnetic moment. The NMR sensitive carbon–13 isotope is only 1.1% in natural abundance. In addition, the sensitivity of ^{13}C is also low (only 1.6% as in ^1H with the same number of isotopes). Thus, so far, all ^{13}C NMR studies in our laboratories are done on mono– and dinucleotides, or homopolymers (1).

Preliminary study on the magnetic shielding effect of the ring–current of purine on ^{13}C atom shows that the chemical shift changes of ^{13}C due to base–base stacking can be calculated from ring–current shielding effect of the purine (15,22,31).

Furthermore, the heterocoupling constants between ^{13}C and ^1H or ^{31}P can add more valuable information about the backbone conformation (1).

C. ^{19}F NMR

Fluorine atom does not exist in natural nucleic acid. However, since ^{19}F is the sole isotope of fluorine and this nucleus has a spin 1/2, as well as relatively high sensitivity (about 83% and ^1H NMR), ^{19}F can be used as a probe. For example, 2'–fluoro–2'–deoxyadenosine and its dimer have been studied and found their conformation is similar to natural dideoxyriboadenosine monophosphate (51). Thus, the ^{19}F signal can be followed in a more complex system such as the helical–coil transition with polyuridylic acid (16).

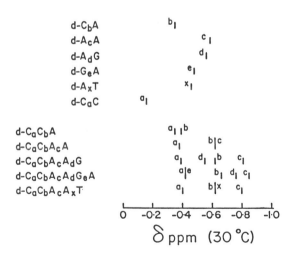

FIG. 32. Comparison of chemical shift of ^{31}P resonance of the dimer to the same dimeric unit within the oligomers, d–C–C–A, d–C–C–A–A, d–C–C–A–A–G, d–C–C–A–A–G–A, and d–C–C–A–A–T. From (13).

FUTURE PROSPECTS

The study of nucleic acid NMR can be divided roughly into two areas: (1) The study on nucleic acid itself, and (2) the study of the interaction between nucleic acid with other molecules, particularly proteins. In the study of nucleic acid itself, in addition to the normal form, or naturally occurring nucleic acid, there is a need to study nucleic acid which has been perturbed by physical binding or covalent linkage with drugs, mutagens, carcinogens, etc. In the study of nucleic acid with other compounds, interaction of proteins such as enzymes, suppressors, and antibodies would be the most common subjects for investigation.

With the advent of the high–field NMR spectrometer equipped with powerful computer, the use of a multiple–pulse technique (such as 2D–COSY and NOESY) has made the ^{1}H NMR a highly developed tool to study nucleic acid, at least the short fragment up to 20 nucleotides in length. The NMR study can certainly supplement the x–ray crystallographic study on one hand, and biochemical studies on the other hand in order to define the structure, the interaction, and to understand the basic mechanism in the biochemical process at the atomic level.

The study of nucleic acid by NMR through other types of nuclei is just beginning. ^{31}P NMR will be most useful in the study of nucleic acid–protein interaction. ^{13}C NMR will be most useful in the study of the dynamic process of nucleic acids. ^{15}N and ^{14}N NMR will be useful to study the hydrogen bonding of base–pairs, particularly the non–Watson–Crick type and finally, ^{17}O NMR will be most useful to study the O–P–O bond in the backbone, as well as for hydrogen bonding involving an oxygen atom. In summary, the study of nucleic acid by different nuclei will provide unique information pertinent to the questions, except for ^{1}H NMR types of NMR studies which will soon be developed to meet this challenge.

REFERENCES

1. Alderfer, J.L. and Ts'o, P.O.P. (1977): Biochemistry 16:2410–2416.
2. Allen, F.H., Bellard, S., Brice, M.D., Cartwright, B.A., Doubleday, A., Higgs, H., Humelink, T., and Watson, B.G. (1979): Acta Crystallog. B35:2331–2343.
3. Altona, C. and Sundaralingam, M. (1972): J. Amer. Chem. Soc. 94:8205–8212.
4. Arnott, S. (1970): Progr. Biophys. Mol. Biol. 21:265–319.
5. Arnott, S., Hukins, D.W.L., and Dover, S.D. (1972): Biochem. Biophys. Res. Commun. 48:1392–1399.
6. Arnott, S., Hukins, D.W.L., Dover, S.D., Fuller, W., and Hodgson, A.R. (1973): J. Mol. Biol. 81:107–122.
7. Bax, A. and Freeman, R. (1981): J. Magn. Reson. 42:164–168; 44:542–561.
8. Blackburn, B.J., Grey, A.A., and Smith, I.C.P. (1970): Can. J. Chem 48:2866–2870.
9. Bloomfield, V.A., Crothers, D., and Tinoco, Jr., I. (1974): Physical Chemistry of Nucleic Acids. Harper and Row, New York.

10. Borer, P.N., Kan, L.-S., and Ts'o, P.O.P. (1975): Biochemistry14:4847–4863.
11. Cantoni, G.L. and Davies, D.R. editors (1971): Procedures in Nucleic Acid Research. Harper and Row, New York.
12. Cheng, D.M., Kan, L.-S., Frechet, D., Ts'o, P.O.P., Uesugi, S., Shida, T., and Ikehara, M. (1984): Biopolymers 23:775–795.
13. Cheng, D.M., Kan, L.-S., Iuorno, V.L., and Ts'o, P.O.P. (1984): Biopolymers 23:575–592.
14. Cheng, D.M., Kan, L.-S., Miller, P.S., Leutzinger, E.E., and Ts'o, P.O.P. (1982): Biopolymers 21:697–701.
15. Cheng, D.M., Kan, L.-S., Ts'o, P.O.P., Giessner-Prettre, C., and Pullman, B. (1980): J. Am. Chem. Soc. 102:525–534.
16. Cheng, D.M., Kan, L.-S., Ts'o, P.O.P., Uesugi, S., Takatsuka, Y., and Ikehara, M. (1983): Biopolymers 22:1427–1444.
17. Crick, F.H.C. and Watson, J.D. (1953): Nature 171:737–738.
18. Crothers, D.M., Cole, P.E., Hilbers, C.W., and Shulman, R.G. (1974): J. Mol. Biol. 87:63–88.
19. Donohue, J. and Trueblood (1960): J. Mol. Biol. 2:363–371.
20. Frechet, D., Cheng, D.M., Kan, L.-S., and Ts'o, P.O.P. (1983):Biochemistry 22:5194–5200.
21. Furberg, S. (1951): Acta Crystallogr. 3:325–331.
22. Giessner-Prettre, C., Pullman, B., Borer, P.N., Kan, L.-S., and Ts'o, P.O.P. (1976): Biopolymers 15:2277–2286.
23. Giessner-Prettre, C., Pullman, B., Prado, F.R., Cheng, D.M., Iuorno, V., and Ts'o, P.O.P. (1984): Biopolymers 23:377–388.
24. Gorenstein, D.G., editor (1984): Phosphorus–31 NMR: Principles and Application. Academic Press, New York.
25. Hall, L.D. (1963): Chem. Ind. (London) 950–951.
26. Kan, L.-S., Borer, P.N., and Ts'o, P.O.P. (1975): Biochemistry14:4864–4869.
27. Kan, L.-S., Chandrasegaran, S., Pulford, S.M., and Miller, P.S. (1983): Proc. Natl. Acad. Sci. USA 80:4263–4265.
28. Kan, L.-S., Cheng, D.M., and Cadet, J. (1982): J. Magn. Resonance 48:86–96.
29. Kan, L.-S., Cheng, D.M., Jayaraman, K., Leutzinger, E.E., Miller, P.S., and Ts'o, P.O.P. (1982): Biochemistry 21:6723–6732.
30. Kan, L.-S., Cheng, D.M., Miller, P.S., Yano, J., and Ts'o, P.O.P. (1980): Biochemistry 19:2122–2132.
31. Kan, L.-S., Kast, J.R., Ts'o, D.Y., and Ts'o, P.O.P. (1979): Biomed. 10:16–28.
32. Kan, L.-S., Ts'o, P.O.P., Sprinzl, M., von der Harr, F., and Cramer, F. (1977): Biochemistry 16:3143–3154.
33. Kan, L.-S. and Ts'o, P.O.P. (1977): Nucleic Acids Res. 4:1633–1647.
34. Karplus, M. (1959): J. Chem. Phys. 30:11–15.
35. Kondo, N.S. and Danyluk, S.S. (1972): J. Am. Chem. Soc. 94:5121–5122.
36. Kondo, N.S., Fang, K.N., Miller, P.S., and Ts'o, P.O.P. (1972): Biochemistry 11:1991–2003.
37. Lakshminarayanan, A.V. and Sasisekharan, V. (1970): Biopolymers 8:475–488; 489–501.
38. Lemieux, R.U., Nagabhushan, T.L., and Paul, B. (1972): Canad. J. Chem. 50:773–776.

39. Macura, S., Huang, Y., Suter, D.S., and Ernst, R.R., (1981): J. Magn. Reson. 43:259–281.
40. Miller, L., Kumar, A., and Ernst, R.R. (1975): J. Chem. Phys. 63:5490–5491.
41. Noggle, J.H. and Schirmer, R.E. (1971): The Nuclear OverhauserEffect: Chemical Applications. Academic Press, New York.
42. Peticolas, W.L. (1981): In: Methods in Structural Molecular Biology, edited by D.B. Davies, W. Saenger, and S.S. Danyluk, pp. 237–266. Plenum Press, London.
43. Quigley, G.J., Seeman, N.C., Wang, A.H.J., Suddath, F.L., and Rich, A. (1975): Nucleic Acids Rev. 2:2329–2341.
44. Schweizer, M.P., Chan, S.I., Helmkamp, G.K., and Ts'o, P.O.P. (1964): Amer. Chem. Soc. 86:696–700.
45. Sundaralingam, M. (1969): Biopolymers 7:821–860.
46. Sundaralingam, M. and Jensen, L.H. (1965): J. Mol. Biol. 13:914–929; 930–943.
47. Tonoco, Jr., I. and C. Bustamente (1981): In: Methods in Structural Molecular Biology, edited by D.B. Davies, W. Saenger, and S.S. Danyluk, pp. 269–305. Plenum Press, London.
48. Ts'o, P.O.P., editor (1974): Basic Principles in Nucleic Acid Chemistry. Academic Press, New York.
49. Ts'o, P.O.P., Kondo, N.S., Schweizer, M.P., and Hollis, D.P. (1969): Biochemistry 8:997–1029.
50. Ts'o, P.O.P., Barrett, J.C., Kan, L.-S., and Miller, P.S. (1973): Ann. New York Acad. Sci. 222:290–306.
51. Uesugi, S., Kaneyasu, T., Imura, J., Ikehara, M., Cheng, D.M.,Kan, L.-S., and Ts'o, P.O.P. (1983): Biopolymers 22:1189–1202.
52. Voet, D. and Rich, A. (1970): Prog. Nucleic Acid Res. Mol. Biol. 10:183–265.
53. Wang, A.H.J., Quigley, G.J., Kolpak, F.J., Crawford, J.L., van Boom, J.H., Van Der Marel, G., and Rich, A. (1979): Nature 282:680–686.

NMR in Biology and Medicine,
edited by Shu Chien and Chien Ho.
Raven Press, New York © 1986.

NMR Studies of Nucleic Acid Structure

Brian R. Reid

*Chemistry and Biochemistry Departments, University of Washington,
Seattle, Washington 98195*

The specificity of DNA recognition by proteins is fundamental to the control of genetic expression. One of the areas of current research in my laboratory is the molecular basis of this sequence specific polymer–polymer interaction at the level of atomic resolution. In these studies we are attempting to use NMR spectroscopy to obtain high–resolution structural information in solution about biologically important DNA sequences such as restriction endonuclease sites, promoter sequences for gene transcription, and operator sequences to which repressors bind to control gene expression. We are also studying the repressor proteins themselves by NMR spectroscopy, but time and space prevent my presenting the protein studies here, and I will restrict myself to studies on the solution structure of DNA.

The research that I will describe requires a talented team of coworkers and I would like to acknowledge at the outset the colleagues and students who did the work, especially Dennis Hare and David Wemmer who performed the NMR experiments, and Shan–Ho Chou and Yim–Foon Lee who synthesized the DNA samples. The experiments I shall describe involve studies of synthetic restriction sequences, promoter sequences and operator sequences of DNA in solution, using two–dimensional NMR spectroscopy (2DNMR).

NMR SPECTROSCOPY OF DNA

The building blocks of DNA are the complementary Watson–Crick base pairs consisting of two deoxyribose sugars and two heterocyclic bases that are hydrogen bonded to each other as shown in Figure 1. Each sugar contains seven aliphatic protons and each base contains three or four aromatic protons. Most NMR experiments are carried out in D_2O solution in which the exchangeable amino and imino base proteons are replaced by deuterons, leaving about 18 protons per base pair. Fortunately, these protons have different chemical shifts and fall into six major spectral regions of the proton NMR spectrum. The 7–8 ppm region contains the aromatic base protons (cytosine and thymine H6, guanine H8, adenine H8 and H2), the 5.2–6.2 ppm region contains the sugar 1'H as well as the cytosine H5, the 4.5–5.0 ppm region contains the sugar 3'H, the 3.7–4.4

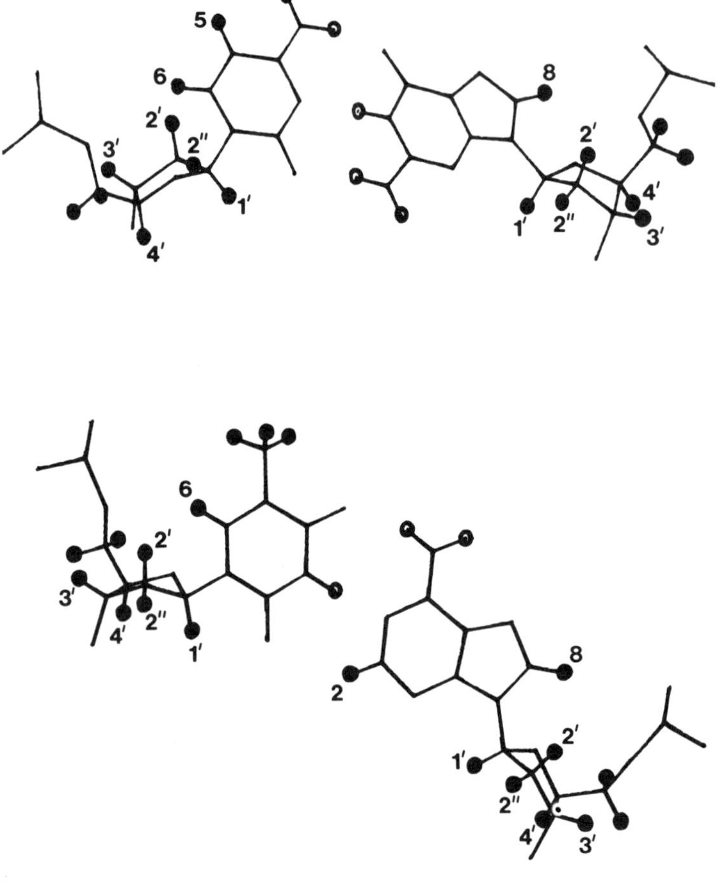

FIG. 1. Watson–Crick base pairs arranged in standard helical geometry. Each deoxyribose contains 7 J–coupled spins. Among the bases, cytosine is the only residue with a pair of vicinal, J–coupled, aromatic protons. Note the spatial proximity of the sugar 2'H to the H6/H8 of its own base.

ppm region contains sugar 4'H, 5'H and 5"H resonances, the 2.0–3.0 region contains the deoxyribose methylene protons (2'H and 2"H), and the methyl groups of thymine are found in the 1–2 ppm region. Thus, the type of proton can usually be determined by visual inspection of the NMR spectrum. More specific information requires a more detailed study of the through–bond J–coupling or the through–space dipolar coupling of these protons. For simple, very small DNA molecules, these couplings can be revealed by classical one–dimensional selective irradiation experiments. However, in a molecule of only 12 base pairs, the spectrum will contain about 200 protons and, even disregarding the problems of overlapping resonances, such experiments would be extremely time consuming. Studies on molecules of this level of complexity require the power and resolution of two–dimensional NMR spectroscopy.

TWO DIMENSIONAL NMR SPECTROSCOPY

Two–dimensional NMR (2DNMR) was originally conceived by Jeener (6) and developed by Ernst, Freeman and their coworkers (1,2,4). In 2DNMR the various spins are frequency–labeled by being allowed to evolve for a short time, t_1, after a 90° pulse. In a NOESY experiment the xy components are next converted to z magnetization by a second 90° pulse followed by a mixing time, t_m, during which magnetization is transferred between proximal spins by cross–relaxation. The system is sampled with a third 90° pulse followed by signal acquisition, and the whole process is repeated for several hundred incremented values of t_1. The NOESY pulse sequence is thus 90° – t_1 – 90° – t_m – 90° – ACQ. After Fourier transformation, the resulting several hundred frequency domain spectra are again Fourier transformed by columns (i.e. as a function of t_1) to generate the 2D NOESY spectrum on two frequency axes. Since each resonance will have the same frequency in ω_1 and ω_2, the resulting auto peaks (the standard 1D spectrum) will lie on a 45° diagonal. However, peaks that exchange magnetization during the mixing time will generate off–diagonal cross peaks that are important in delineating pairs of proximal, dipolar coupled, protons. The analogous COSY 2DNMR experiment involves a 90° – t_1 – 90° – ACQ pulse sequence, in which magnetization transfer is mediated by through–bond J–coupling, i.e. pairs of protons separated by 2,3 or 4 bonds are identified by their cross peaks. The extensive J–coupling between protons on a single sugar residue can be identified in the COSY spectrum, whereas through–space couplings between protons on adjacent residues are revealed in the NOESY spectrum.

2D NMR OF DNA

The COSY and NOESY spectra of the Eco R1 sequence d(CGCGAATTCGCG)$_2$ are shown in Figure 2. In the COSY spectrum, the expected couplings between 1'H and 2',2"H, between 2',2"H and 3'H, and between 3'H and 4'H are revealed by cross peaks at the intersections of the appropriate spectral regions. Furthermore, cytosine is the only base in DNA that contains two protons on adjacent carbon atoms: the strong aromatic H6–H5 couplings from the 7 ppm region to the 5.5 ppm region thus identify the four cytosines in the molecule, and even the two thymines can be identified from their four–bond couplings to methyl resonances around 1.5 ppm. The remaining purine protons are, by elimination, at the lower field 8 ppm end of the aromatic resonances. The main function of the COSY map is that, for any given 1'H, a set of other protons can be identified from their J–coupling as belonging to the same sugar. Thus, one can segregate the sugar protons into 12 discrete spin systems.

The NOESY map serves to orient each residue in the DNA chain by means of inter–residue dipolar coupling (the NOE). For instance, the most upfield aromatic resonance, at 7.1 ppm is obviously the H6 of either T7 or T8 by virtue of its 4–bond COSY coupling to the upfield methyl resonance

CGCGAATTCGCG

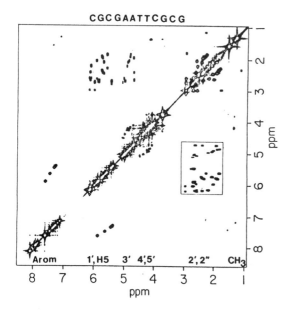

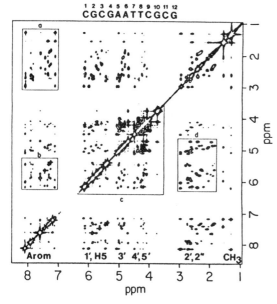

FIG. 2. The COSY (top) and NOESY (bottom) spectra of the Eco R1 sequence d(CGCGAATTCGCG). The COSY spectrum cross peaks reveal the extensive J–coupling between the 1',2',2",3', and 4' protons in a single sugar spin system, as well as the strong H5–H6 coupling in the 4 cytosines. The NOESY spectrum reveals the large number of dipolar couplings from a given proton to proximal protons on the same residue and on adjacent residues.

at 1.2 ppm. The fact that the 1.2 ppm methyl exhibits an NOE to an adjacent purine H8 at 8.1 ppm establishes that it is T7 rather than T8 (T8 has pyrimidines on either side) and thus assigns the most upfield aromatic proton (7.1 ppm) as the H6 of T7. With the foothold of this specific assignment, one can now ask what types of protons are within NOE distance (< ca. 5 Å) of this thymine H6. Looking along the NOESY row at 7.1 ppm, one sees NOE cross peaks to two 1' protons, two 3' protons, two protons in the 4',5',5" region, three protons in the 2',2" region, and two methyl groups (the 1.5 ppm methyl is from T8). The proximity of two 1'H resonances is especially informative in that it allows the preceding sugar (in this case A6) to be identified. The fact that each aromatic H6 (or purine H8) exhibits NOEs to two 1'H resonances (its own and the preceding sugar) and vice versa, constitutes a sequential connectivity path along the DNA chain that can be traced in this region of the spectrum (box b). This sequential zig–zag trace is shown in expanded view in Figure 3.

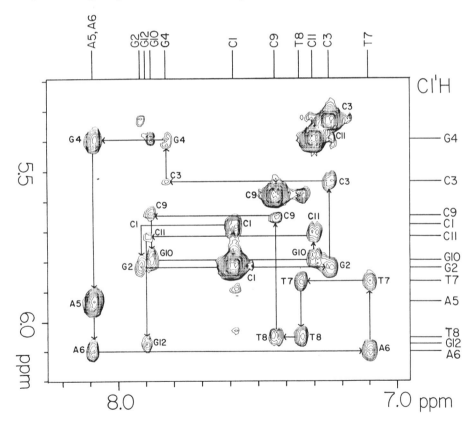

FIG. 3. Expansion of the aromatic – 1'H cross peaks (box b) of Fig. 2. Each aromatic H6/H8 (vertical columns) shows two cross peaks, one to its own 1'H and one to the preceding (5'–side) 1'H. Similarly each 1'H (horizontal rows) shows cross peaks to two base protons.

Once the 1'H of the preceding residue has been identified, the other protons of this sugar can be easily identified as components of the J–coupled spin system of that sugar in the COSY spectrum. However, it should be emphasized that this is by no means the only sequential connectivity path through the DNA chain. The right–handed nature of B–DNA results in the appearance of detectable NOEs from the aromatic H6/H8 to its own 2'H and 2"H, the preceding 2"H, and often the preceding 2'H. Thus, three or four NOEs are often observed in the 2–3 ppm region, and constitute an alternative path of connectivity down the chain. These sequential assignment pathways in DNA NOESY spectra were first used to assign DNA NOESY spectra by Hare et al. (5) and Scheek et al. (9) in 1983. The correct identification of the preceding 2"H can be corroborated by consulting the COSY map and verifying that it is indeed J–coupled to the preceding 1'H as determined by the first connectivity path. Alternatively, the identities of the preceding sugar 2'H and 2"H can be checked from their dipolar coupling to 1'H of this sugar (i.e. box d in the NOESY map): the trans 1'H–2'H NOEs are usually weaker than the gauche 1'H–2"H NOEs. Thus, the COSY/NOESY data are highly redundant, with many independent corroborations, leading to a very high level of confidence in the assignments. Typically, the 100–200 protons in a DNA sequence of 10–15 base pairs can be uniquely assigned in a few hours of analysis.

STRUCTURAL ANALYSIS

Up to this point, the NOEs in the NOESY map have been used only qualitatively to establish the presence or absence of a proximal proton. However, the data can be re–analyzed in terms of NOE intensities in order to derive structural information. For instance, in the "idealized" B–DNA structure obtained from fiber diffraction coordinates, the distance from an aromatic H6/H8 to its own 1'H should be the same as the distance to the preceding 1'H to within 0.2 A. Thus, the two 1'H cross peaks from a given H6/H8 should be quite similar in intensity. This appears to be true for T8, T7, A6 and A5 (see Figure 3). However, in the case of G4 the H8 NOE to its own 1'H and to the 1'H of C3 are much weaker. An obvious question is can such variations in cross peak intensity be interpreted quantitatively to yield accurate structural information. The answer appears to be a qualified "yes", provided some precautions are taken.

In DNA molecules of around 12 base pairs in size (mol. wt. ca. 7,500), the molecules cannot tumble fast enough in solution to generate fluctuating fields at the Larmour frequency. Hence, zero quantum cross relaxation (mutual spin–spin flipping) dominates the longitudinal relaxation process. This cross relaxation has the form

$$R_1 = \gamma^4 \hbar^2 \tau_c / 10 r^6$$

and hence the distance, r, between two protons should be related to the amount of z–magnetization transferred in a given time. However, if a proximal spin B becomes "hot" by virtue of its proximity to spin A, it can now further transfer magnetization to more distant spins C and D which would thus appear to be close to spin A. This process is termed "spin diffusion" and has been treated in detail by Kalk and Berendsen (7): it is a serious problem in attempting to derive distance information in polymers. Typical NOE build up rates for close and intermediate protons are shown graphically in Figure 4, as well as a typical spin diffusion second order effect to a more distant proton. In general, the effects of spin diffusion can be eliminated by determining the NOE build up rate using several different mixing times, or else one can use a sufficiently short mixing time such that second order effects are not yet detectable. A further potential problem in this approach to measuring distances is the possibility of differential local motion i.e. all proton pairs may not share the same correlation time and hence would transfer magnetization at different rates, even if the distances were the same. However, from preliminary experiments we have carried out, this does not appear to be a serious problem. We have repeated the NOESY experiment of Figure 2 (which was taken with a 300 msec mixing time) using a 100 msec mixing time and scaled the aromatic –1'H and aromatic–2',2"H intensities (box b and box a) to the fixed H5–H6 distance of a cytidine (the strong cross peaks in box b). The NOE distances from several aromatic H6/H8 protons to the surrounding 1'H, 2'H protons were then calculated from the corresponding cross peak intensities and compared to these distances in the crystal structure of the molecule (3). Some results are summarized in Table 1. The NMR distances and the x–ray distances agree to within about 0.5 Å

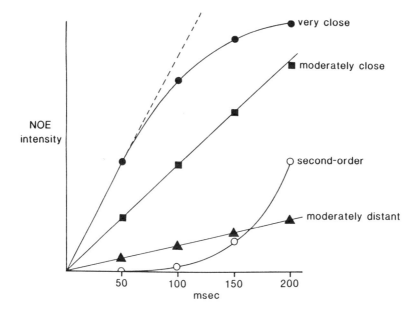

FIG. 4. Typical rates of NOE build up by cross–saturation for very close, moderately close, and moderately distant proton pairs. Note that more distant, second order, spin–diffusion effects show a lag period. At short mixing times in the 50–100 msec range, only direct first order effects are detected.

TABLE 1.   Interproton distances in d(CGCGAATTCGCG)$_2$ obtained from
0.1 sec NOESY peaks by scaling intensities to the fixed
cytosine H5–H6 distance (2,4A).

	Distance					
Proton	T7 1'	T6 1'	T7 2'	T7 2"	T6 2'	T6 2"
T7 H6	3.6	3.3	2.7	3.5	2.9	2.8
	(3.6)	(3.6)	(2.5)	(3.7)	(3.6)	(2.6)
	G4 1'	C3 1'	G4 2'	G4 2"	C3 2'	C3 2"
G4 H8	3.7	>4	2.5	2.9	3.3	3.1
	(3.7)	(4.7)	(2.2)	(3.4)	(2.5)	(2.8)

Values in parentheses refer to the corresponding distances observed in
the crystal structure of d(CGCGAATTCGCG)$_2$. See (3).

suggesting that local motion does not seriously compromise this method of
probing molecular structure: the results also yield an estimate of the
precision of this approach.

SIZE LIMITS OF THE NMR METHOD

We have carried out studies similar to those described above on
promoter DNA sequences containing 12 base pairs without symmetry i.e. 24
unique residues rather than 12 (10). In this case each strand is a distinct
entity and must be traced separately as shown in Figure 5. Nevertheless,
unique assignments can be made using the same strategies as before (10).
Even larger molecules such as operators can be assigned by this approach.
Figure 6 shows the COSY and NOESY spectra of the OR3 operator
sequence containing 34 unique residues. Assignments have been made and
structural comparisons have been made between the wildtype sequence and
a mutant operator (12). Using phase–sensitive methods to improve the line
shape of the cross peaks, it appears that at field strengths of 500 MHz,
molecules in the 20–30 base pair range can be assigned.

NON–DUPLEX DNA STRUCTURES

Given the relative ease with which standard B–DNA NMR spectra can
now be assigned, an obvious question is can these techniques be used to
reveal the existence of interesting atypical DNA structures in solution?
We have recently studied a variation of the d(CGCGAATTCGCT) molecule
that has the d(CGCGTATACGCG) sequence. The aromatic–1'H NOE
connectivities for this sequence are shown in Figure 7. At 0.1–0.2 M NaCl,
a typical B–DNA sequential connectivity trace can be followed, but several

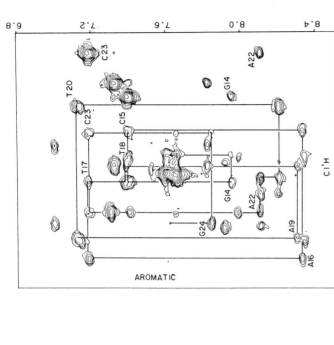

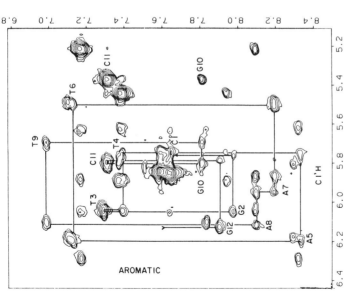

FIG. 5. The aromatic – 1'H NOESY connectivities for the non–symmetrical Pribnow promoter sequence d(CGTTATAATGCG) + d(CGGCATTATAACG). Note that the 1–12 strand (left) and the 13–24 strand (right) have independent connectivity networks.

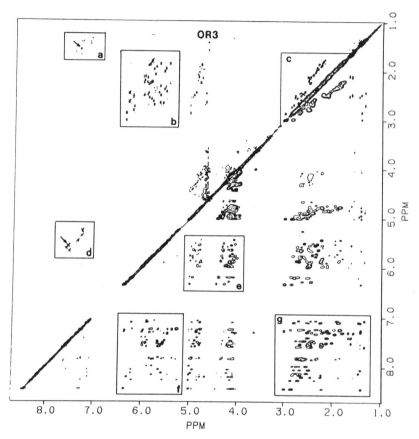

FIG. 6. The COSY (upper left) and NOESY (lower right) spectra of the bacteriophage lambda OR3 operator DNA sequence containing 34 nucleotides. Sequential connectivities down each strand can be traced in boxes f and g (12).

extra anomalous cross peaks are also detected, suggesting the existence of a second structure in solution (11). The existence of two structures in solution can easily be seen from the one–dimensional spectra of the methyl resonances of the two thymine residues, shown in Figure 8. At 0.3 M NaCl the molecule exhibits all the normal NOE connectivities and is presumably in the regular B–DNA form. However, between 0.05 M and 0.2 M NaCl a new structure, in equilibrium with the B–DNA duplex, is formed in solution. Below 10 mM NaCl this new structure predominates. Selective saturation recovery experiments on this new structure revealed that it had T_1 values that were twice as long as those of the duplex, suggesting that it was only one half the molecular weight of the duplex

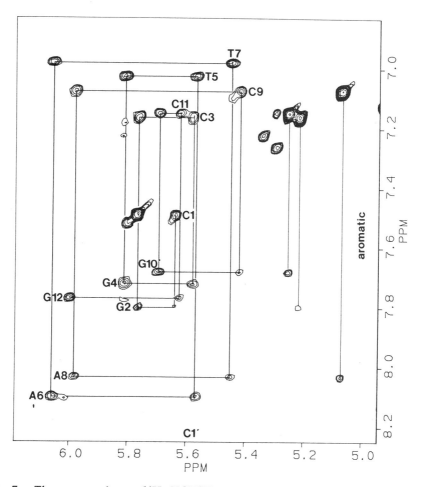

FIG. 7. The aromatic – 1'H NOESY connectivities for the sequence d(CGCGTATACGCG) at intermediate ionic strength. Note the additional unconnected cross peaks from the hairpin conformation in the upper right corner.

i.e. only one strand. Furthermore, studies in H_2O solution revealed that only four base pairs (GC pairs) were formed, strongly indicating a hairpin structure in which residues 1–4 and 9–12 formed base pairs. The duplex–hairpin population ratio was also found to be temperature dependent, from which a van't Hoff transition enthalpy of 30 kcal/mole could be calculated. The transition enthalpy for converting each hairpin strand to the denatured single strand form was also ca. 30 kcal/mole, in good agreement with the duplex–random coil enthalpy of 90 kcal/mole for sequences such as d(CGCGAATTCGCT) and d(CGCGTATACGCG) estimated by standard methods (8).

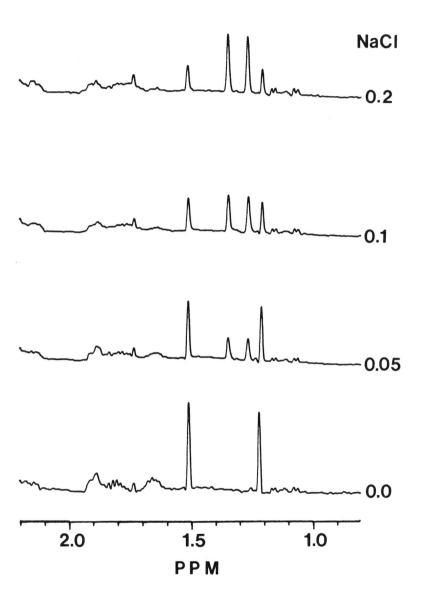

FIG. 8. The one–dimensional NMR spectrum of the methyl region of d(CGCGTATACGCG) at various ionic strengths. Note the splitting of the two thymine methyl resonances indicating two conformations of the molecule at intermediate ionic strength.

In terms of the kinetics of interconversion, the rate of the duplex–hairpin conversion was conveniently measurable on the NMR time–scale by direct transfer of saturation. Thus, the forward rate constant could be determined at various temperatures, from which the Arrhenius activation energy of 50 kcal/mole for hairpin formation could be calculated (11). The fact that this activation energy is far less than the transition enthalpy for single strand formation, effectively precludes any mechanism for hairpin formation involving sequential end–fraying to form a single–stranded intermediate. The only reasonable alternative is a central bulging of the four AT pairs followed by a propagating cruciform structure as shown in Figure 9.

Such structures are of potential biological importance and the structure of the hairpin loop is of some interest. Dennis Hare, a current member of my laboratory, became interested in such loops and has investigated the hairpin structure d(CGCGTTTTCGCG) in solution by 2DNMR. Using time–dependent NOESY spectra, several hundred distances between assigned protons were determined. Compared to standard B–DNA, several "anomalous" NOEs were observed between protons not usually found in close proximity. An example is shown in Figure 10 where the methyl group

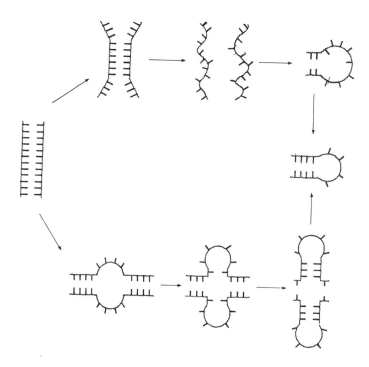

FIG. 9. Possible models for duplex–hairpin interconversion in d(CGCGTATACGCG). The observed activation energy and transition enthalpy effectively eliminate the single–stranded upper route and strongly favor the cruciform lower route.

of T7 was found to be close to the 1' protons of T5, T6 and T7. Such unexpected NOEs are very valuable in defining the spatial orientation of the loop residues in this hairpin. Using all of these constraints to create a distance file, Dr. Hare wrote a computer algorithm to embed this multi–dimensional problem in three–dimensional space. The resulting structure was refined to minimize the differences from the original NOE distance constraints, resulting in the structure shown in Figure 11. The generation of such structures directly from solution data requires considerable amounts of computer time (1–2 days) but offer the important advantage of being able to analyze structures that cannot be crystallized. We are continuing studies on other hairpin loop structures in solution using these methods.

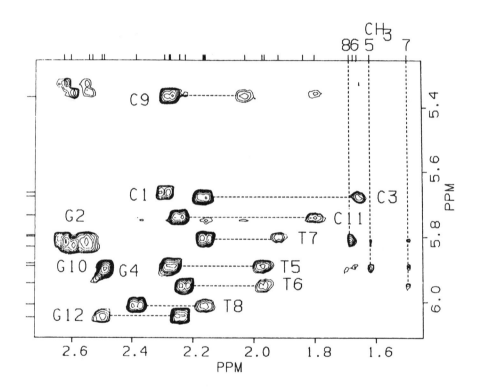

FIG. 10. The NOESY cross peaks in the 1'H to 2',2" Me region of the d(CGCGTTTTCGCG) hairpin. Note the cross peaks from the T7 methyl resonance to the 1' protons of T5, T6 and T7.

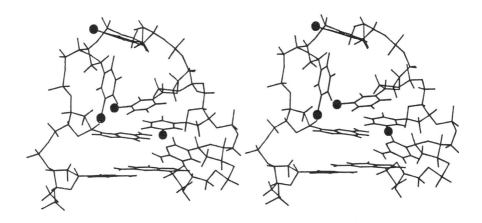

FIG. 11. Stereo view of a partially refined hairpin loop structure in solution. This structure was created by embedding all the NOESY distance constraints in 3–space and refining the structure to minimize the experimentally observed distances (D.R. Hare, unpublished).

REFERENCES

1. Aue, W.P., Bartholdi, E., and Ernst, R.R. (1976): <u>J. Chem. Phys.</u> 64:2229–2246.
2. Bachmann, P., Aue, W.P., Muller, L., and Ernst, R.R. (1977): <u>J. Magn. Reson.</u> 28:29–39.
3. Dickerson, R.E. (1983): <u>J. Mol. Biol.</u> 166:419–441.
4. Freeman, R. and Morris, G.A. (1979): <u>Bull. Magn. Reson.</u> 1:5–26.
5. Hare, D.R., Wemmer, D.E., Chou, S.H., Drobny, G., and Reid, B.R. (1983): <u>J. Mol. Biol.</u> 171:319–336.
6. Jeener, J. (1971): Abst. Ampere Summer School. Basko Poljie, Yugoslavia.
7. Kalk, A. and Berendsen, H.J.C. (1976): <u>J. Magn. Reson.</u> 24:343–366.
8. Marky, L.A., Blumenfeld, K.S., Kozlowski, S., and Breslauer, K.J. (1983): <u>Biopolymers</u> 22:1247–1257.
9. Scheek, R.M., Russo, N., Boelens, R., Kaptein, R., and van Boom, J.H. (1983): <u>J. Amer. Chem. Soc.</u> 105:2914–2916.
10. Wemmer, D.E., Chou, S.H., Hare, D.R., and Reid, B.R. (1984): <u>Biochemistry</u> 23:2262–2268.
11. Wemmer, D.E., Chou, S.H., Hare, D.R., and Reid, B.R. (1985): <u>Nucleic Acids Res.</u> 13:3755–3772.
12. Wemmer, D.E., Chou, S.H., and Reid, B.R. (1984): <u>J. Mol. Biol.</u> 180:41–60.

III. NMR IMAGING

NMR in Biology and Medicine,
edited by Shu Chien and Chien Ho.
Raven Press, New York © 1986.

New Directions in NMR Zeugmatographic Imaging

Paul C. Lauterbur*

Departments of Chemistry and Radiology, State University of New York at Stony Brook, Stony Brook, New York 11794

INTRODUCTION

Nuclear magnetic resonance (NMR) imaging and spectroscopy are continuing to evolve rapidly, especially for medical applications (2). The use of the zeugmatographic (5) principle for imaging offers many opportunities for devising new techniques. When these are combined with the many clever and subtle NMR spectroscopic techniques that have been, and continue to be, developed, a great richness of possibilities becomes available. In this review, two recent directions that NMR imaging has taken will be described. Spectroscopic imaging (or zeugmatographic spectroscopy) is not new. It was first demonstrated many years ago (7), and a number of alternative methods have since been invented (2). The recent method (1,8) to be reviewed here is unusual in the clarity with which it illustrates the close connection between imaging and spectroscopy and the opportunities it offers for carrying out technically straightforward investigations with essentially standard NMR spectrometers. Another development that was first discussed in general (5) and more specific (3,9,10) terms some time ago is microscopic imaging. The more recent work to be reviewed here has produced the first such images of useful quality (4,6) as well as a detailed analysis of both theoretical and experimental aspects of their formation (4).

SPECTROSCOPIC IMAGING BY PROJECTION RECONSTRUCTION

A linear magnetic field gradient shifts the frequency of an NMR signal from a particular point in space by an amount proportional to the distance of that point from the null plane, where the gradient field vanishes and only the homogeneous magnetic field remains. If the nuclei are initially

---

* present address: Departments of Medical Information Science and Chemistry, University of Illinois, 1307 West Park, Urbana, Illinois 61801, U.S.A.

on resonance in the homogeneous field, a simple geometrical construction shows that the frequency offsets in a set of differently–oriented gradients correspond to projections of that point if all of the null planes intesect in a line (in two dimensions) or a point (in three dimensions). The same diagram will show that signals initially displaced in frequency by an amount independent of the direction of the magnetic field gradient do not correspond to a set of projections, because all of their projections back into the image are tangent to a circle centered at the location at which they would have intersected in the absence of the initial frequency displacement. Within that circle the back–projected signal intensity vanishes. If the projections have been filtered before back–projection to give a true image the inner region even has a negative intensity (4). Such behavior suggests that projection reconstruction of images from signals containing more than one spectral line is impossible, because only one line could be properly centered and the others would give rise to misleading artifacts. That is ordinarily true, but an extension of the idea of projection reconstruction into an additional dimension resolves the difficulty (1,8). Figure 1 indicates the concept underlying the method. For an object with only one spatial dimension, the complete spectroscopic image can be represented as a set of intensitites associated with a two–dimensional pseudo–object, as shown in Figure 1. It is clear that the two orthogonal projections shown there are simply the image and the spectrum of the original one–dimensional object. The image would be obtained by

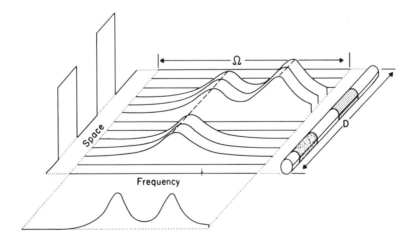

FIG. 1. The cylinder on the right represents a one–dimensional object with length D, composed of material whose NMR signals lie within a spectral bandwidth Ω. The NMR signal intensities in a 2–dimensional pseudo–object defined by the coordinates D and Ω may be regarded as a surface obtained by tracing the spectra associated with each point along the cylinder. The projection onto the spatial axis is the integrated NMR signal from each such point, and the projection along the frequency axis is just the NMR spectrum of the object in a homogeneous magnetic field.

the imposition of an infinitely large magnetic field gradient, along the spatial axis, which would entirely suppress the spectral information. In practice, of course, a gradient would need be only large enough so that the scaled spectra would fall within a single picture element and be unresolved in the image. It can be shown (8) that the use of smaller gradients corresponds to viewing the pseudo–object at other angles θ, given by θ = tan^{-1} (γGD/Ω), where θ is the angle between the frequency axis and the projection direction, γ is the magnetogyric ratio, G is the magnetic field gradient strength, and D and Ω are defined in Figure 1. The width of each measured projection must be multiplied by cos θ to obtain the corresponding view of the pseudo–object. When that is done, data obtained with a fixed gradient direction but different gradient strengths correspond precisely to projections of the pseudo–object at angles calculated from the above equation. The same equations and computer programs used to reconstruct purely spatial images of real objects from their projections can therefore be used to reconstruct spectroscopic images. Simulations of this procedure for objects similar to that in Figure 1 have verified its validity (8). The pure spatial projection at 90° cannot be obtained experimentaly, but there are reconstruction algorithms that can be used, with some success, when some of the projections are missing, and one of these has produced reasonable results in simulations (8).

THREE DIMENSIONAL PROJECTION RECONSTRUCTION
OF A SPECTROSCOPIC IMAGE FROM EXPERIMENTAL DATA

Experiments designed to test this new technique have been carried out on a test object made from two plastic containers 75 mm high, 25 mm wide, and 14 mm thick (1). One contained water and the other acetic acid, and the proton NMR signals were obtained at 4 MHz using a modification (1) of a 0.094 mT whole–body imaging system (12). Magnetic field gradient components were applied along the directions of the height and width of the object, but the third component was not used. In the absence of chemical shifts, the resulting rotation of the gradient in a plane would have led to the reconstruction of a two–dimensional projection of the three–dimensional object. In this experiment, the third dimension was reserved for the intrinsic frequency axis along which the spectra were to be reconstructed. To obtain projections of the three–dimensional pseudo–object, the magnitude of the magnetic field gradient was changed through a series of steps, from about 3μT/m to about 500 μT/m, for each spatial direction. The total number of gradients was 1891, distributed over a complete set of angles chosen to give uniform coverage while avoiding the 90° case that would require an infinite gradient. For each gradient the free induction decay was recorded after a radiofrequency pulse, and the reconstruction was carried out, on the appropriately–scaled projections, using the hybrid algorithm (11) and a 64x64x64 array. Figure 2 shows the experimental image as projections on planes perpendicular to the frequency axis. All 64 reconstructed planes are projected on the spatial plane in Figure 2a to give an image undistorted by the presence of three distinct peaks in the spectrum. In Figure 2b is shown the sum of 8 planes centered on the frequency of the water resonance, Figure 2c shows the sum of 5 planes containing the carboxylic proton resonance, and the location of the methyl protons is shown by the sum of 6 planes displayed in Figure 2d.

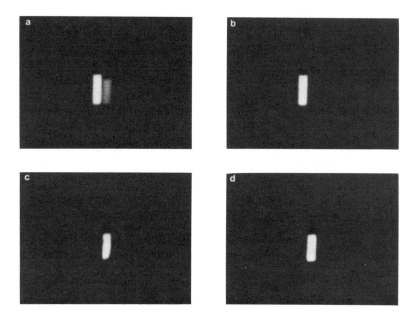

FIG. 2. Spatial images of the two–dimensional test object obtained from the three–dimensional spectroscopic reconstruction, as described in the text: (a) the total proton image, (b) the water proton image, (c) the acetic acid carboxylic proton image, and (d) the acetic acid methyl proton image.

It can be seen that the spectroscopic image has been completely resolved, even at the very low proton NMR frequency of 4MHz, and that images free of chemical shift artifacts can be recovered. Very little modification is required to enable any NMR spectrometer, even a CW instrument, to obtain such images. The gradients may be generated by existing linear shim coils with appropriate current controls. Because they do not need to be changed rapidly, eddy currents and other transients are not important, and static gradients make it possible to use free induction decay signals as well as spin echoes, and to image materials with transverse relaxation rates too rapid for the usual spin–echo methods to be practical.

Four–dimensional imaging, to give complete spectroscopic images of three–dimensional objects, should be possible by straightforward extensions of such experiments and reconstruction algorithms, although the data acquisition may take an impractically long time for some applications if the usual procedures are employed.

IMAGING OF MICROSCOPIC OBJECTS

It has been realized for many years that the resolution in an NMR image is usually limited by the signal–to–noise ratio (10). Although that ratio can be improved, for a given observed volume element, as the receiver coil diminishes in size, the signal from a volume element proportional in size to the coil decreases rapidly, as the inverse cube of its linear dimensions. Eventually, for a signal comparable to that from a 10 μm cube of water or similar material (10^{-15} m^3), useful imaging begins to become impractical. Careful experimental investigations of the possibility of developing an NMR microscope have only recently been begun, however (4). To obtain the images shown below, a special probe was built for use in a 2.1 tesla iron–core electromagnet. The radiofrequency coil was wound on a 1.7 mm diameter glass capillary tube. Outside it, but within the probe, were placed gradient coils less than 10 mm in diameter, so as to give large gradients over a small region with reasonable currents. Preliminary experiments have been carried out at 90 MHz on water proton signals in test samples and small biological objects. An example of some of the results obtained on a 1 mm snail are shown in Figure 3 (4).

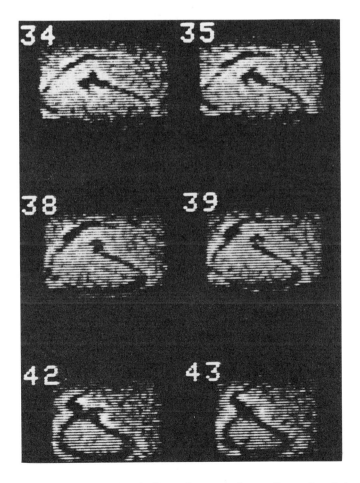

FIG. 3. Selected longitudinal slices from a three–dimensional image of a small snail. Each slice, a single plane from the reconstructed image, is about 1 mm across and 2 mm high, although the image is compressed, as described in the text.

A three–dimensional volume image was generated by projection reconstruction on a 64x64x64 array. The gradient component along the vertical axis was smaller than the other two, giving an anisotropic image with the long axis compressed, so that the volume elements were about 20x20x70 μm in size. The selected 20 μm thick slices shown clearly display the internal architecture of the dense shell against background of the signals from the inner tissues and the water in which the animal was immersed. With improvements in resolution and contrast it may become possible to see soft tissue anatomy, as is done in medical imaging, and perhaps even some detail at the cellular level.

ACKNOWLEDGMENTS

This work was supported in part by Grant No. CA15300, awarded by the National Cancer Institute, DHHS, by Grant No. HL19851, awarded by the National Heart, Lung and Blood Institute, DHHS, and by National Science Foundation Grant No. PCM800629–A01.

REFERENCES

1. Bernardo, M.L., Jr., Lauterbur, P.C., and Hedges, L.K. (1985): J. Magn. Res. 61:168–174.
2. Budinger, T.F., and Lauterbur, P.C. (1984): Science 226:288–298.
3. Grannell, P.K., and Mansfield, P. (1975): Phys. Med. Biol., 20:477–482.
4. Hedges, L.K. (1984): Ph.D. Dissertation, Dept. of Physics, State Univ. of New York at Stony Brook, Stony Brook, New York.
5. Lauterbur, P.C. (1973): Nature (London) 242:190–191.
6. Lauterbur, P.C.: Proceedings of the 1984 Takeda Science Foundation Symposium on Bioscience (in press).
7. Lauterbur, P.C., Kramer, D.M., House, W.V., Jr., and Chen, C.–N. (1975): J. Am. Chem. Soc. 97:6866–6868.
8. Lauterbur, P.C., Levin, D.N., and Marr, R.B. (1984): J. Magn. Reson., 59:536–541.
9. Mansfield, P. and Grannell, P.K. (1975): Phys. Rev. B., 12:3618–3634.
10. Mansfield, P., and Morris, P.G. (1982): NMR Imaging in Biomedicine, Supplement 2 to Advances in Magnetic Resonance, edited by J.S. Waugh, pp. 191–216. Academic Press, New York.
11. Marr, R.B., Chen, C.–N., and Lauterbur, P.C. (1981): In Mathematical Aspects of Computerized Tomography, Vol. 8, edited by G.J. Herman and F. Natterer, pp. 225–240. Springer Verlag, Berlin.
12 Simon, H.E. (1981): Applications of Optical Imaging in Medicine IX, Proc. Soc. Photo–Optical Instrum. Engin., 273:41–49.

NMR in Biology and Medicine,
edited by Shu Chien and Chien Ho.
Raven Press, New York © 1986.

Magnetic Resonance Imaging of the Musculoskeletal System

Harry K. Genant, *,**, Michael L. Richardson, †,
Thurman Gillespy III, *, Clyde A. Helms, * Neil I. Chafetz, *

*Department of Radiology, ** Department of Orthopaedic Surgery, University of California
San Francisco, California 94143, † University of Washington School of Medicine,
Seattle, Washington 98195*

Magnetic resonance imaging (MRI) is a technique of potential value in assessing the musculoskeletal system. In the following review, we relate our experience with MRI in healthy subjects and in patients with musculoskeletal disease (6,8,9).

There are several features of MRI that make it particularly attractive for musculoskeletal imaging: (1) the superior soft–tissue contrast resolution of MRI relative to that of computed tomography (CT); (2) the ability of MRI to image the body directly in the sagittal and coronal planes, as well as the axial plane; (3) the ability to vary the level of contrast between tissues by manipulating the MRI pulse–sequence parameters; (4) the lack of artifacts from beam–hardening effects; and (5) the capacity to image in the presence of metallic hardware. Magnetic resonance imaging of the musculoskeletal system currently appears to hold greatest promise in five major areas: (1) the noninvasive imaging of the spine and disc disease; (2) the early detection of osteonecrosis of the femoral head; (3) the evaluation of the extent and tissue characteristics of musculoskeletal tumors; (4) the assessment of focal and diffuse marrow–replacing processes; and (5) the depiction of articular and periarticular structures. In the remainder of this review, we will discuss our experience with these and other disorders.

TECHNICAL CONSIDERATIONS

All subjects included in this review were examined at the University of California, San Francisco using a Diasonics MT/S Imaging System. This system consists of a 0.5–T superconducting magnet that is currently operated at a field strength of 0.35T. To date, we have acquired all of our images by using the spin echo (SE) technique. This technique yields gray scale anatomic images in which the intensity of a tissue is a complex function of the T_1, T_2, and spin density of that tissue. The relative magnetic resonance gray scale for body tissues in general is shown in Table I and Figure 1. Representative T_1 and T_2 values for various musculoskeletal tissues are shown in Table II. Although cortical bone returns little signal, the high intensity signal of the adjacent marrow and the medium intensity muscle signal more than compensate for this, making visualization of the cortical bone between them generally quite easy. By varying the pulse sequence used, one can markedly vary the contrast between two tissues. The eight different pulse sequences currently available on our system are summarized in Table III.

Table I. Magnetic Resonance Spin–echo Gray Scale
in Descending Order of Brightness*

Fat

Marrow and cancellous bone

Nucleus pulposus

Brain and spinal cord

Viscera

Muscle

Fluid–filled cavities

Ligaments and tendons

Blood vessels with rapid flow

Compact bone

Air

---

* The brighter the image, the shorter is the T_1 and/or the longer is the T_2. The darker the image, the longer is the T_1 and/or the shorter is the T_2 and/or the lower is the proton density.

FIG. 1A,B (On next page). Sagittal magnetic resonance (MR) images of the head and neck (A: top) and thoracic spine (B: bottom) showing the range of gray scale values seen in human tissue with spin echo (SE) techniques.

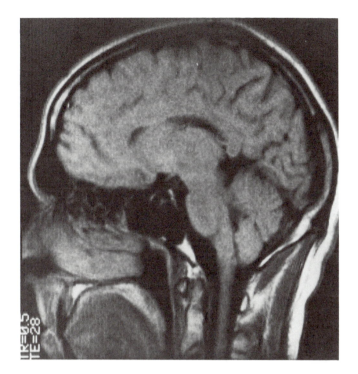

FIG. 1A

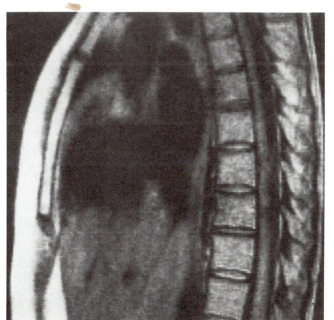

FIG. 1B

Table II. T_1 and T_2 Values Obtained from Normal Tissues

Tissue	T_1 (msec±S.D.)	T_2 (msec±S.D.)	No. of samples
Muscle	541 ± 141	35 ± 6	13
Subcutaneous fat	218 ± 68	61 ± 18	12
Vertebral marrow	420 ± 112	50 ± 12	16
Nucleus pulposus	1078 ± 396	65 ± 17	22
Ligament–tendon	864 ± 206	107 ± 16	3

TABLE III. Spin–echo Imaging Sequences

TR (msec)	TE (msec)	No. of Sections	Imaging Time (min)
500	28,56	5	4.5
1000	28,56	10	9.0
1500	28,56	15	13.5
2000	28,56	20	18.0

FIG. 2A–C (on next page). Three sagittal SE MR images in the same subject. (A) with the short TR (TR, 0.5 sec; TE, 28 msec) sequence, the thecal contents are isointense with the annulus fibrosis. It would be difficult to exclude disc bulging or subtle herniation with this image. (B) with a long TR (TR, 2 sec; TE, 28 msec) sequence, the thecal contents become brighter than the annulus. Note the normally bright signal seen in the nucleus pulposus. (C) with both a long TR and second echo (TR, 2 sec; TE, 56 msec) sequence, the thecal sac becomes even brighter, making it easy to exclude disc bulging or herniation on this image.

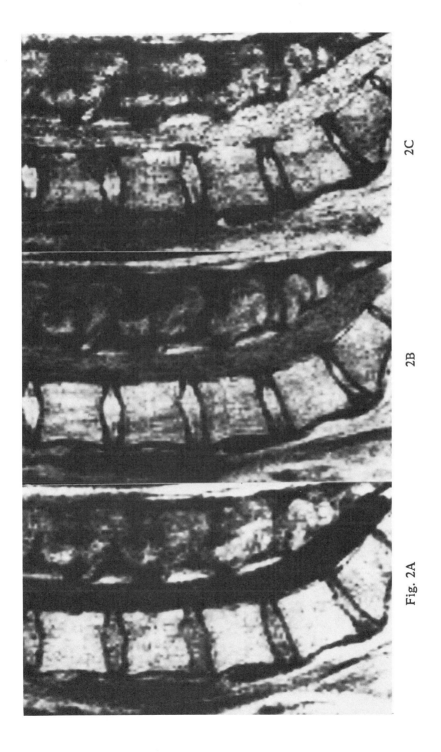

Fig. 2A   2B   2C

MAGNETIC RESONANCE IMAGING OF THE SPINE

Axial imaging of the spine by CT has been an important tool in the evaluation of back pain, and the spatial resolution of axial CT currently exceeds that of axial MRI. MRI, however, has soft tissue contrast resolution superior to that of CT and has the ability to vary this contrast by merely changing the pulse sequence (Fig. 2). Magnetic resonance imaging also adds the ability to directly image large regions of the spine in sagittal and coronal planes while maintaining high image quality (4) (Fig. 3).

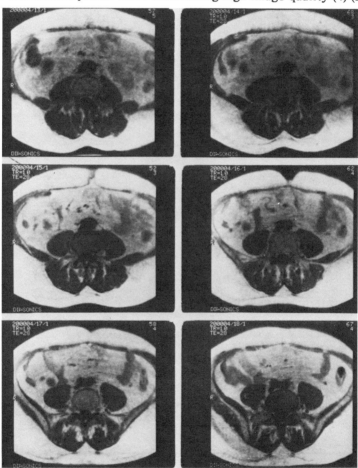

FIG. 3. A series of axial MR images (TR, 1 sec; TE, 28 msec) of the lower lumbar spine demonstrate the normal anatomic structures and relationships that provide the basis for interpretation of studies in patients with low back pain syndrome. The thecal sac and nerve roots are delineated by the surrounding high–intensity epidural and perineural fat. Ligamentum flavum, annulus fibrosis, and articular facets have an extremely low intensity signal.

Many of the same spinal abnormalities seen with conventional radiography, myelography, or CT are also demonstrated on MRI studies. These include narrowing of the intervertebral disc space, disc bulges and herniations, spondylolisthesis, and osteophytosis. However, some findings are unique to MRI. One example of this is the decreased signal intensity observed in degeneration of the nucleus pulposus. When a herniated disc is treated by chemonucleolysis, the treated disc decreases in size and gradually loses signal intensity. With the ability of MRI to distinguish annulus fibrosis from nucleus pulposus, one can demonstrate the herniation

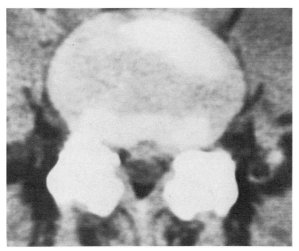

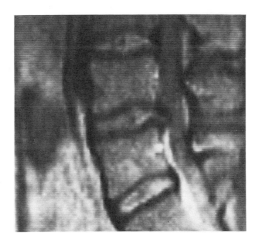

FIG. 4A,B. Axial computed tomographic (CT) image (A: Top) and sagittal SE (TR, 1 sec; TE, 28 msec) MR image (B: Bottom) of the lumbar spine show a large focal central disc protrusion at L4–5. The MR image demonstrates discrete herniation with protrusion of the nucleus pulposus through the annulus fibers posteriorly.

of nuclear material through the annular fibers (Fig. 4). Lateral disc herniation can also be demonstrated with MRI. The exceptional soft–tissue contrast resolution of MRI enables one to differentiate tissues that would appear isodense on a corresponding CT image. For example, the spinal cord can easily be seen within the thecal sac in the thoracic spine (Fig. 1B). We have had little experience with MRI of postoperative fibrosis but are optimistic that it may prove useful in differentiating fibrosis from thecal sac or recurrent disc disease (Fig. 5).

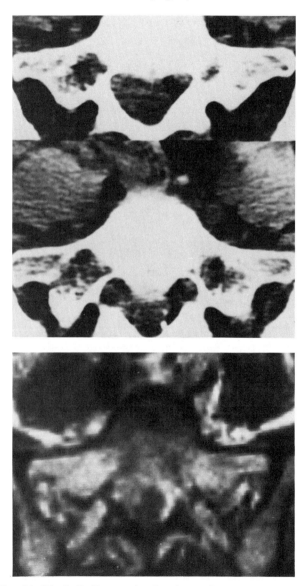

Fig. 5A (Top), B (Bottom). See legends on next page.

There are still several problems to be solved before MRI supplants CT as the study of choice for spinal disease. For example, in its present configuration our MRI instrument cannot produce slices thinner that 7 mm, and when slices are scanned in a multislice mode, a gap of 3 to 4 mm is left unimaged between adjacent slices. These problems make it possible to miss subtle disc abnormalities. When high–resolution images of cortical bone are required, such as in the work–up of spinal stenosis or complex spinal fractures, CT is still necessary.

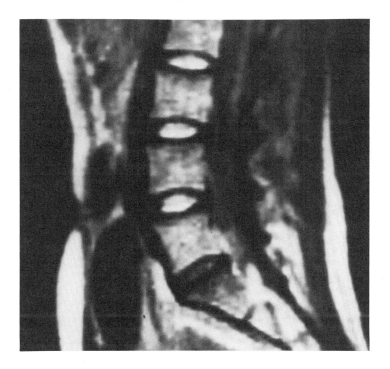

FIG. 5C

FIG. 5A–C. (A: Top of previous page) Two axial CT images at L5–S1 in a postdiscectomy patient demonstrate a mass effect in the right lateral recess of S1 with x–ray attenuation comparable to that of the thecal sac. (B: Bottom of previous page) Axial (TR, 2 sec; TE, 28 msec) MR image of; the same level shows that the mass in the mass in the right lateral recess has an intermediate signal intensity and is easily distinguished from the thecal sac. (C: This page) Right parasagittal MR image demonstrates and intermediate signal intensity mass at L5–S1, which at surgery was found to be a large focus of postoperative scar tissue. The absence of interfacet artifacts (commonly seen with CT) and the ability to distinctly image postoperative scar tissue are promising potential features of MR imaging in the lumbar spine.

MAGNETIC RESONANCE IMAGING OF THE HIP JOINTS

In general, standard radiography and CT are satisfactory for imaging most disorders of the hip joints. However, there is currently no ideal noninvasive method for the early detection of osteonecrosis (avascular necrosis or aseptic necrosis) of the femoral head. Radionuclide scintigraphy of the hips has been helpful in the early diagnosis of osteonecrosis in many patients. However, this technique is not specific for osteonecrosis, and scans must be interpreted with knowledge of the radiographic and clinical findings. It is important to diagnose osteonecrosis before irreversible changes have occurred, because surgery, such as a core decompression procedure, may be able to prevent the progression of osteonecrosis if performed sufficiently early. Intraosseous manometry and phlebography may be able to give early evidence of osteonecrosis but require the insertion of a trocar into the marrow of the femoral neck. To avoid what would be a painful procedure, these tests are generally done under general anesthesia.

Magnetic resonance imaging is capable of showing the normal and abnormal anatomy of the hips in exquisite detail (Fig. 6). Early evidence indicates that MRI of the hip may be useful in the early detection of osteonecrosis (8). In the 24 patients with osteonecrosis that we have studied with MRI to be at least as sensitive as CT in demonstrating changes in the femoral head and far better than conventional radiography (Fig. 7). In all patients with radiographic evidence of avascular necrosis, MR images have shown inhomogeneous loss of the normal high–intensity signal in the femoral head. In several patients with minimal or no radiographic changes, definite abnormalities were found on the MR images, such as mottled or scalloped areas of low intensity within the femoral head. However, our experience is still not large, and a prospective study comparing MRI, CT, radionuclide scintigraphy, and perhaps intraosseous manometry/phlebography in patients at high risk for osteonecrosis (e.g., steroid use and lupus erythematosus) will be necessary to assess the usefulness of MRI in this disease.

We believe that MRI may also be useful in the preoperative evaluation of patients with known osteonecrosis. The transtrochanteric rotational osteotomy is currently performed in our center for osteonecrosis. The rationale for this procedure is as follows: The weight–bearing portion of the femoral head is usually the portion of the femoral head most severely affected by osteonecrosis and the posterior non–weight–bearing portion is often relatively unaffected. In this procedure a transtrochanteric osteotomy is performed and the unaffected portion of the head is rotated up into a weight–bearing position. Currently, standard radiographs are used by orthopedists to judge whether or not an adequate amount of unaffected femoral head remains to warrant the procedure. Both MRI and CT may prove useful in better defining the extent of involvement of the head by osteonecrosis, particularly when axial, coronal, and sagittal images are combined.

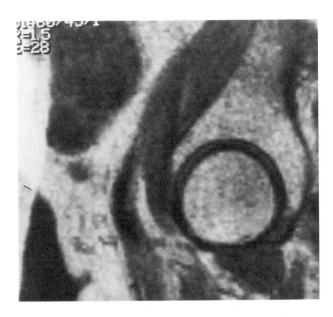

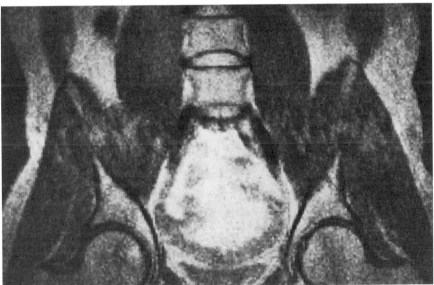

FIG. 6A–B. Sagittal (A: Top) and coronal (B: Bottom) MR imaging through normal hips. Note the excellent delineation of normal osseous, articular, ligamentous and muscular.

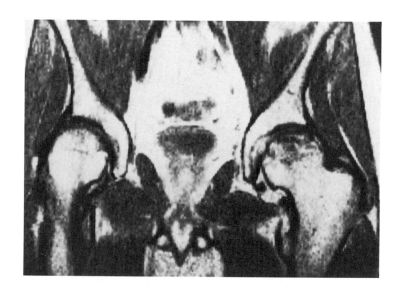

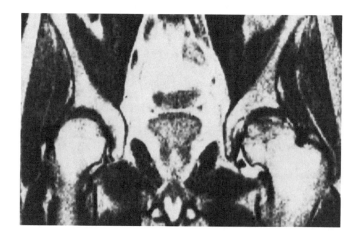

FIG. 7A (Top), B (Bottom). See legends on next page.

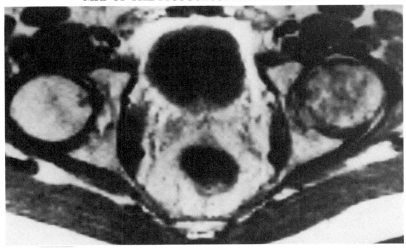

FIG. 7C

FIG. 7A–C. Spin echo coronal MR images of the hips with two pulse sequences: (a) TR, 2 sec; TE, 28 msec and (b) TR, 2 sec; TE, 56 msec. (A,B) These images demonstrate osteonecrosis of the left femoral head with mottled low intensity signal and deformity of the articular surface of the femoral head. Capsular distention from a joint effusion is also illustrated. Note the relative increase in signal in joint fluid compared with muscle between the first and second echo images. (C) Axial MR image (TR, 1.5 sec; TE, 28 msec) of the same subject also shows inhomogeneous loss of signal in the left femoral head and a joint effusion.

MAGNETIC RESONANCE IMAGING OF MUSCULOSKELETAL TUMORS

With its exceptional soft–tissue contrast resolution, MRI offers useful anatomic information on many tumors that is not available with other imaging methods (Fig. 8). We have found MRI most useful in the work–up of primary malignant musculoskeletal tumors, such as fibrosarcoma, malignant giant cell tumor (Fig. 9), and chordoma. Magnetic resonance imaging accurately represents the boundaries of these tumors (1,12) and is superior to CT in displaying the tissue planes between neoplasm, muscle, marrow, and subcutaneous fat.

By analysis of the T_1, T_2 and spin density of tumors and of the surrounding normal muscle and fat, it is possible to optimize the contrast between two given tissues in an SE image. In all the tumors we have imaged so far, optimum contrast between tumor and normal tissue was achieved by means of a scanning protocol containing both short (0.5 sec) and long (2 sec) values of TR (11). In general, images obtained at intermediate values of TR (1 or 1.5 sec on our instrument) displayed inferior contrast between tumor and normal tissue.

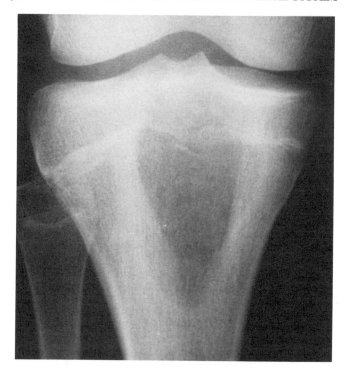

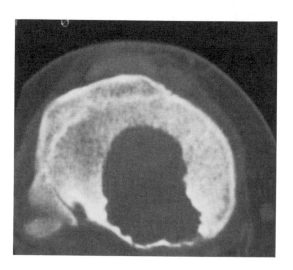

FIG. 8A (Top), B (Bottom). See legends under Fig. 8E.

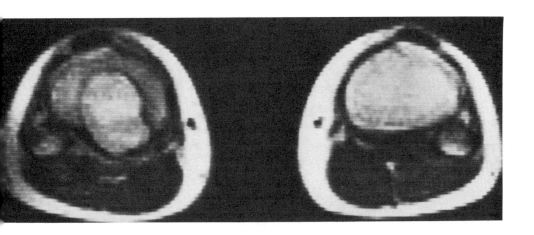

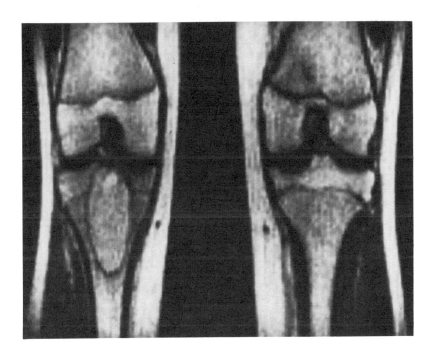

FIG. 8C (Top), D (Bottom). See legends under Fig. 8E.

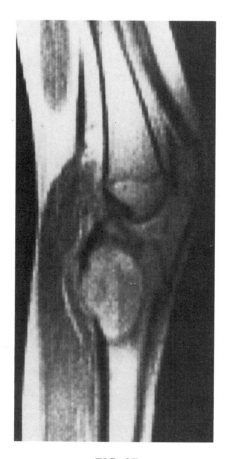

FIG. 8E

FIG. 8A–E. (A) Conventional radiograph demonstrates a lytic aneurysmal bone cyst involving the proximal tibia of an adolescent. (B) Computed tomogram demonstrates the lytic destruction of cancellous bone and mild expansion of the posterior cortex. The aneurysmal bone cyst is approximately isodense with muscle. (C–E): The axial (C), coronal (D), and sagittal (E) MR (TR, 1.5 sec; TE, 28 msec) images demonstrate a relatively high intensity signal of the aneurysmal bone cyst in contrast to adjacent marrow, muscle, and blood vessel. The improved density discrimination with MRI may enhance the diagnostic capabilities, while the multiplanar capability may facilitate surgical management.

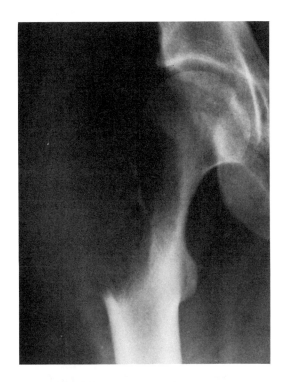

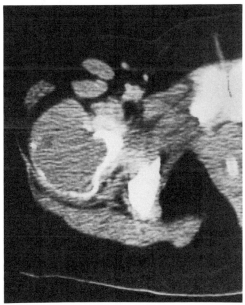

FIG. 9A (Top), B (Bottom). See legends on next page.

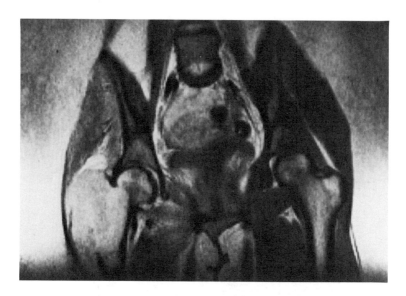

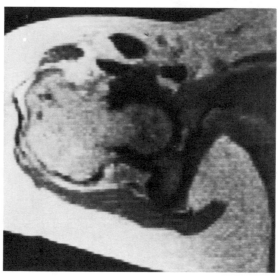

FIG. 9A–D. (A: top of previous page) Conventional radiograph demonstrates a lytic tumor of the proximal femur with an associated soft tissue mass representing an atypical giant–cell tumor. (B: bottom of previous page) Computed tomogram demonstrates the soft–tissue component, which has attenuation characteristics similar to those of muscle and vessels. Coronal (C: Top of this page) and axial (D: bottom of this page) SE MR images (TR, 2 sec; TE, 28 msec) demonstrate the intra- and extraosseous extent of the neoplasm and differentiate it readily from muscle, tendons, vessels, and fat. The right gluteal musculature demonstrates an alteration in signal intensity that may be related to edema and/or atrophy with fatty replacement, or both.

MARROW REPLACEMENT DISORDERS

An intense, uniform, homogeneous signal is seen in normal bone marrow with MRI. Therefore, MRI has the potential to be extremely useful in the evaluation of marrow–based disorders, such as osteomyelitis (5) certain anemias (2) (Fig. 10A), and malignancies such as leukemia, lymphoma, and metastasis to marrow (3) (Fig. 10B). It may also be useful in assessing marrow changes secondary to therapy in these disorders.

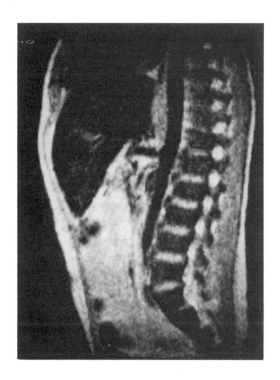

FIG. 10A. See legends on next page.

ARTICULAR DISORDERS

Current MRI technology permits the visualization of many soft–tissue structures, such as tendons and perhaps, more importantly, articular cartilage (7). We have studied several patients with osteochondritis dissecans of the talus with MRI and have been able to demonstrate the gross changes in this disorder (Fig. 11). In the knee the cruciate ligaments and articular cartilage can clearly be seen (Fig. 12). Meniscal cartilage is more difficult to image successfully, because of the difficulty in differentiating meniscal cartilage form articular cartilage and subchondral bone. Magnetic resonance imaging currently has the ability to demonstrate joint effusions. It may one day be possible to distinguish inflammatory from noninflammatory effusions with MRI. When surface coils and other improvements in spatial resolution become widely available, MRI may be useful in the study of injuries to the ligaments and tendons of the shoulder, hip, knee, and ankle and may be able to supplant arthrography and tenography in the larger joints.

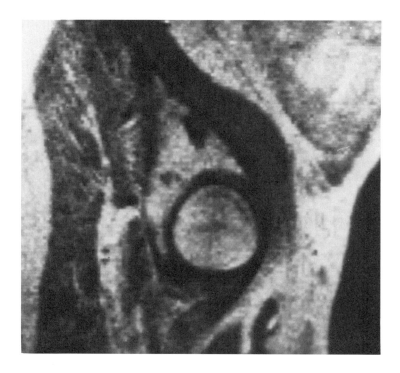

FIG. 10B

FIG. 10A–B. (A) Patient with β–thalassemia with excessive marrow iron deposition. This sagittal SE (TR, 1 sec; TE, 28 msec) MR image of the thoracolumbar spine shows dramatic loss of the normal high intensity signal from the vertebral medullary cavities. Reproduced, with permission from Brasch et al. (9). (B) Parasagittal MR image (TR, 1.5 sec; TE, 28 msec) of the right hip demonstrates several mottled, low–intensity foci in the supraacetabular marrow of the ilium, representing metastatic prostatic carcinoma.

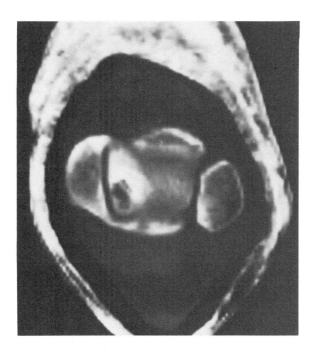

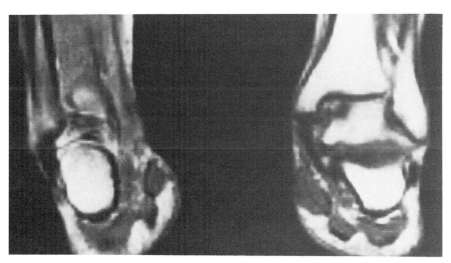

FIG. 11A–B. (A: Top) Axial CT scan through the dome of the left talus showing a focal area of osteochondritis dissecans in the medial dome. (B: Bottom) Coronal MR image (TR, 1.5 sec; TE, 28 msec) showing the same area of osteochondritis dissecans. Note that although the patient has the same plaster cast about the left ankle as shown in the CT image, it cannot be seen in the MR image.

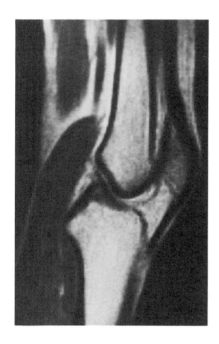

FIG. 12A–B. Sagittal SE (TR, 2 sec; TE, 28 msec) image of the knee of a normal volunteer. The quadriceps tendon, the patellar ligament, and the anterior and posterior cruciate ligaments are well defined.

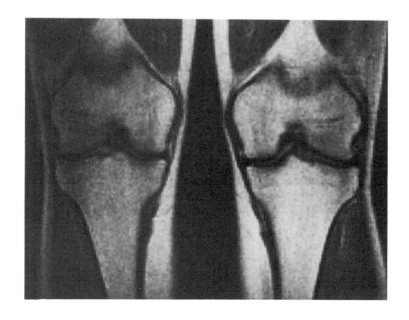

MISCELLANEOUS MUSCULOSKELETAL APPLICATIONS OF MAGNETIC RESONANCE IMAGING

Magnetic resonance imaging has several miscellaneous applications in the musculoskeletal system. (1) In patients with non–ferromagnetic joint prostheses, MRI may one day be useful in the study of loosening or infection. (2) In patients with spinal trauma, MRI may one day be useful in assessing ligamentous integrity and may enable better predictions as to the stability of a particular injury. (3) Because of the lack of ionizing radiation, MRI may prove extremely useful in examining musculoskeletal disorders in pregnant patients. (4) Magnetic resonance imaging has the potential to be useful in the study of muscle disorders, such as atrophy (Fig. 9C), muscular dystrophy (10), and other myopathies. (5) It may prove useful in the study of fracture healing, particularly once imaging can be combined with spectroscopy for the study of local biochemical changes during healing.

SUMMARY

Magnetic resonance imaging is currently a complementary technique to CT in the examination of the spine, the hip, and musculoskeletal tumors. In some cases, it provides diagnostic information not available with any other modality, including CT. Magnetic resonance imaging has the potential to be extremely useful in the assessment of various marrow–based disorders and may someday obviate the need for contrast–aided studies of ligaments, tendons, and cartilage.

REFERENCES

1. Brady, T.J., Gebhardt, M.C., Pykett, I.L., Buonanno, F.S., Newhouse, J.H., Burt, C.T., Smith, R.J., Mankin, H.J., Kistler, J.P., Goldman, M.R., Hinshaw, W.S., and Pohost, G.M. (1982): Radiology 144:549–552.
2. Brasch, R.C., Wesbey G.E., Gooding, C.A., and Koerper, M.A. (1984): Radiology 150:761–771.
3. Cohen, M.D., Klatte, E.C., Bachner, R., Smith, J.A., Martin–Simmerman, P., Carr, B.E., Provisor, A.J., Weetman, R.M., Coates, T., Siddiqui, A., Weisman, S.J., Berkow, R., McKenna, S., and McGuire, W.A. (1984): Radiology 151:715–718.
4. Chafetz, N.I., Genant, H.K., Moon, K.L. Jr., Helms, C.A., and Morris, J.W. (1983): Am. J. Roentgenol. 141:1153–1156.
5. Fletcher, B.D., Scoles, P.V., and Nelson, A.D. (1984): Radiology 150:57–60.
6. Genant, H.K., Moon, K.L. Jr., Heller, M., Chafetz, N.I., and Helms, C.A. (1983): In: Spine Update 1984: Perspectives in Radiology, Orthopaedic Surgery, and Neurosurgery, edited by H.K. Genant, pp. 359–398, Radiology Research and Education Foundation, San Francisco, CA.

7. Kean, D.M., Worthington, B.S., Preston, B.J., Roebuck, E.J., McKim–Thomas, H., Hawkes, R.C., Holland, G.N., and Moore, W.S. (1983): Br. J. Radiol. 56:355–364.
8. Moon, K.L. Jr., Genant, H.K., Helms, C.A. Chafetz, N.I., Crooks, L.E., and Kaufman, L. (1983): Radiology 147:161–171.
9. Moon, K.L. Jr., Genant, H.K., Davis, P.L., Chafetz, N.I., Helms, C.A., Morris, J.M., Rodrigo, J.J., Jergesen, H.E., Brasch, R.C., and Bovill, E.G., Jr. (1983): J. Orthop. Res. 1:101–114.
10. Newman, R.J., Bore, P.J., Chan, L., Gadian, D.G., Styles, P., Taylor, D., and Radda, G.K. (1982): Br. Med. J. Clin. Res. 284:1072–1074.
11. Richardson, M.L., Amparo, E.G., Helms, C.A., et al (1984): Program of the Annual Meeting of the Association of University Radiologists. Abstract 128.
12. Steiner, R.M., Falke, T., Taminiau, A., et al (1984): Program of the Annual Meeting of the American Roentgen Ray Society. Abstract 139.

NMR in Biology and Medicine,
edited by Shu Chien and Chien Ho.
Raven Press, New York © 1986.

Magnetic Resonance of the Cardiovascular System

Ralph J. Alfidi

Department of Radiology, Case–Western Reserve University, Cleveland Ohio 44106

INTRODUCTION

Magnetic resonance is a rapidly developing field (1,2,3), and equipment can become obsolete in a short time. For example, at Case–Western Reserve, the 3–kGauss magnet installed in April 1982 has already been replaced with one with a higher field strength, which will allow us to do better head and body magnetic resonance imaging (MRI).

The greatest diagnostic challenges in MRI are: (a) early detection of neoplasm, (b) intermediate large scale detection of cardiovascular diseases, (c) detection of degenerative diseases, e.g. Alzheimer's disease, and (d) detection of multicellular–level tissue injury or change. The advantages and limitations in clinical MRI are listed in Table I. With respect to the body, the slow acquisition time causes significant limitations in spatial resolution. Throughput is a problem in MRI. Currently, when we look through a series of pulse frequencies, the patient may be in the magnet for 1 to 1 1/2 hours. Although there is a great deal of enthusiasm in MRI, there may be some overdoing. Scrutiny in various institutions has not substantiated the earlier claim that MRI is tissue specific. Recently a monoclonal antibody developed by Dr. Cheung (4) from neuroblastoma of nude mice has been tagged with a high degree of specificity. We have used this monoclonal antibody to show human tumors in the cavernium and femurs with very little background counts. It may be possible to label monoclonal antibodies with paramagnetic substances such as gadolinium DPTA. The question is whether a sufficient amount of the substance will gain access to allow MRI.

We are interested in the cardiovascular system because there is a significant number of coronary heart disease. In 1984, some 4,600,000 patients had either heart attack or angina in the United States. There were 559,000 heart attack death; 350,000 of them died before reaching the hospital. Asymptomatic coronary heart disease patients with potentially lethal situations are not detected. Stress tests and nuclear medicine techniques are not reliable, and the gold standard is still coronary angiography. Hence an important goal is to develop a technique which will allow us to detect these asymptomatic cases on an out–patient survey basis, perhaps as a part of the physical examination.

Table I. Advantages and Limitations in Clinical MRI

MRI Advantages (Clinical)

1. No known hazard
2. Virtually unlimited technique parameters
3. Rapidly expanding field with many potential directions
4. Flow void phenomenon–Blood flow quantification possible

MRI Limitations (Clinical)

I.   Data Acquisition Time – Slow
     a. Gating – C.R.
     b. New technology (Acquisition Time) – E.P.
     c. New Magnet design – New coil designs

II. Spatial Resolution
     a. Improvement necessary to compete with U.S., C.T.
     b. Angiographic applications
        1. Improved surface coil technology
        2. Improved region of interest–technology
        3. Other

III. Throughput

IV. Tissue Characterization

MAGNETIC RESONANCE IMAGING OF VASCULAR SYSTEM

An ideal vascular imaging system should have the following characteristcs. These include a good spatial resolution, a good contrast resolution, the ability to differentiate the flowing blood in the artery lumen, the absence of physical hazards, being non–invasive, requiring no catheterization or contrast medium, the ability to visualize the vessel in three dimensions, a low cost, and a high patient throughput. In addition, the ideal cardiac MRI technique should allow a rapid data requisition, have a spatial resolution of 0.5 mm or better, and permit the survey of a susceptible patient population.

One of the reasons why MRI is interesting for studying the cardiovascular system is the flow–void phemomenon, i.e. the absence of signal in a flowing fluid in a variety of pulse sequences in MRI. In Figure 1, a large arteriovenous malformation of the brain is seen as a black structure because there is no flow, while the vessel with flow is white, with 100% contrast. MRI is a tomographic technique. In addition to axial images (Figures 2 and 3), MR can also be used to obtain sagittal and coronal images (Figures 4 and 5). One can visualize the carotid arteries, subclavian arteries, ventricular chambers, coronary arteries, pulmonary artery, abdominal aorta and vena cava (5).

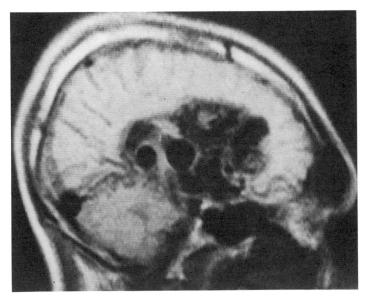

FIG. 1. MR showing a large arteriovenous malformation in the brain.

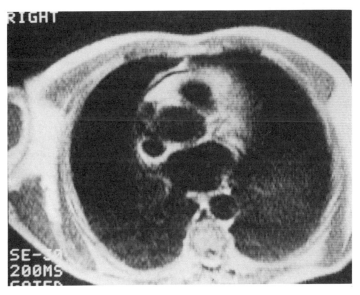

FIG. 2. Axial MR scan at the level of the left atrium (LA). Left main (arrow) and circumflex coronary arteries are arising from ascending aorta. ECG cardiac gating. From (5).

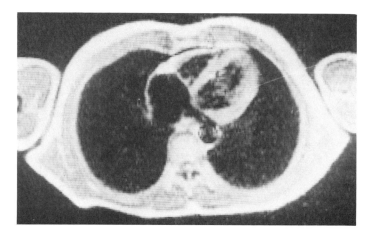

FIG. 3. Axial MR scan below the left atrium demonstrating three chambers and the tricuspid valve (arrow). Combined arterial pulse and respiratory gating. From (5).

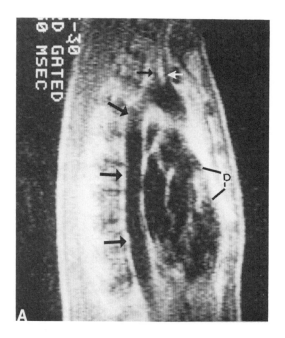

FIG. 4. Sagittal MR scan trom a normal subject with cardiac gating, demonstrating the various vessels in three slices. A (above), left of midline: the aortic arch and descending aorta (black arrows), carotid artery (small white arrow), and subclavian arteries (small arrow), and pulmonary trunk (P). B (next page), Midline: the right pulmonary artery (large arrow) and trachea (small arrows). C (next page), Right of midline: the right main bronchus (large arrow), right pulmonary artery (small arrow), superior vena cava (S), and inferior vena cava (curved arrow). From (6).

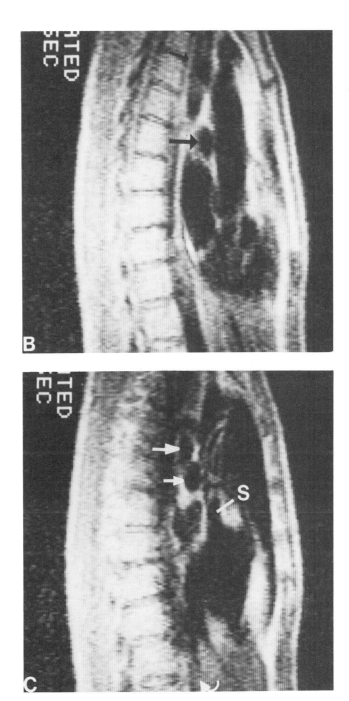

FIG. 4. B (top) and C (bottom). See preceding page for legends.

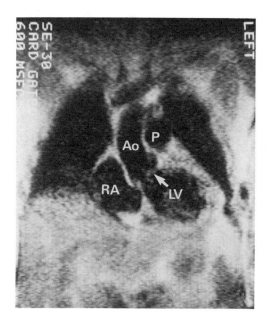

FIG. 5. Coronal MR scan demonstrating right atrium (RA), left ventricle (LV), ascending aorta (Ao), main pulmonary artery (P), and aortic valve (arrow). ECG cardiac gating. From (5).

GATING OF CARDIAC AND RESPIRATORY MOVEMENTS

Although MRI can give good images of the cardiovascular system, there are some problems. In some respects, MRI is like photography. A long imaging time will result in blurring of moving objects. Heart undergoes systole and diastole; respiration cycles cause more severe problems. MRI of a phantom moved by 1 cm at an oscillation frequency of 12 cycles/min ($\simeq$ normal respiratory rate) showed not only a diminution of the clarity of the structures in comparison to the static image, but also the production of harmonics as artefacts to distort the image. Experimental studies on dogs also showed that stoppage of breathing by intravenous curare led to a marked increase in the clarity of the image. Therefore, respiratory movements are a major problem in the quality of MRI. As the organs move, partial volume averaging causes deterioration of image and affects the values of T_1 and T_2 determined on these organs.

Gating of Cardiac Movement

When a heart is in motion, one can barely see the ventricular chambers and the septum. Figures 2–5 were obtained by cardiac gating, i.e. synchronization of data acquisition with arterial pulse or, better yet, with electrocardiogram (7); this leads to a marked improvement in image. We use a radio–telemetry system to obtain the gated image, which obviates the interference problems. The cardiac valves, cardiac chambers, interventricular septum, and even some stumps of the papillary muscle can be visualized.

Combination of Cardiac and Respiratory Gating

When MRI is performed in a subject during breathing, one sees poor definitions of the edge of the diaphragm, the portal system, and structures within the cardiac silhouette. Respiratory gating (correlation of deep expiration with data acquisition) alone improved the edge definition of the diaphragm, but the cardiac structures are still poorly defined. Cardiac gating alone leads to an improvement of the definition of the cardiac wall, but the liver and the portal system again have a diminished image quality. Combined cardiac and respiratory gating yields a much more superior picture (Figure 6). One clearly sees the portal system, the edge of the liver, the diaphragm, and the cardiac structures.

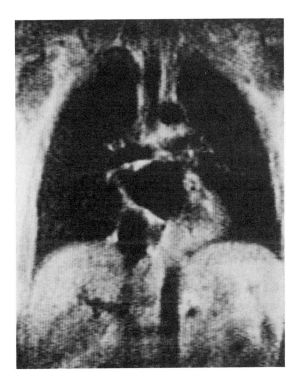

FIG. 6. Coronal MR scan at the level of the left atrium (LA). Note the sharpness of the diaphragm. Combined arterial pulse and respiratory gating. From (5).

The gating process, however, causes an increase in data acquisition time. Cardiac gating alone doubles the data acquisition time, and combined cardiac and respiratory gating triples it. In general, cardiac gating is not a problem, whereas respiratory gating is. In a static structure, e.g. the brain, infarct can be easily detected on MRI, and infarcts in the heart can only be detected with appropriate gating.

MAGNETIC RESONANCE IMAGING IN VASCULAR DISORDERS

Figure 7 shows the abdominal aorta, the iliac branches, the vena cava with its iliac branches, and renal arteries in a normal subject. Figure 8 shows a dissecting aortic aneurysm, which can now be diagnosed very well by MRI, and the gold standard is again angiogram (Figure 8A). One can see the various portions of the dissecting aneurysm, the true and false lumen and the septum in between them.

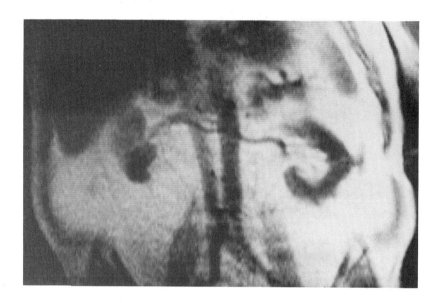

FIG. 7. MR scan showing the abdominal aorta, the iliac branches, the vena cava with its iliac branches, and renal arteries in a normal subject.

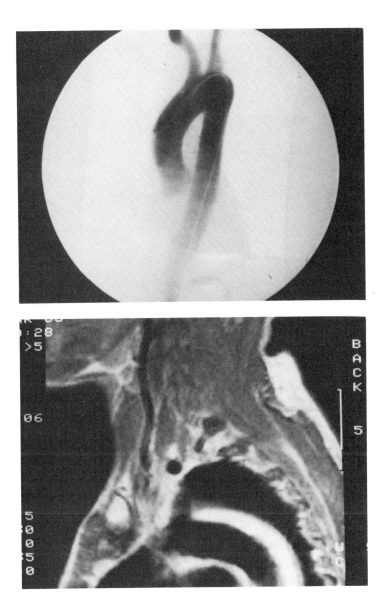

FIG. 8. Angiogram (top) and MR scan (bottom) showing a dissecting aortic aneurysm.

In a subacute endocarditis patient with blood stream infection, one can see on angiogram the escape of the injected contrast medium from a false channel in the wall to a mycotic aneurysm, which can be seen on CT or MRI in various planes of projection (Figure 9).

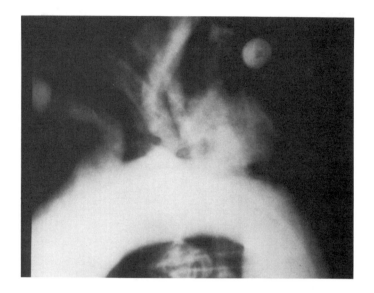

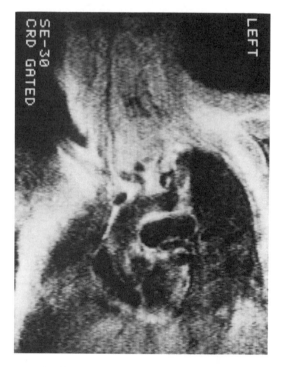

FIG. 9. Angiogram (top) and MR scan (bottom) showing the escape of the injected contrast medium from a false channel in the wall to a mycotic aneurysm in a subacute endocarditis patient.

The MRI in Figure 10 shows the blockade of the external iliac artery branch on one side, as indicated by the presence of only one black hole on that side, instead of the two black holes, one for artery and the other for vein, on the normal side. Figures 11A and 11B show the MR scan and angiogram, respectively, of an aorta with arteriosclerotic plaques along the lateral wall.

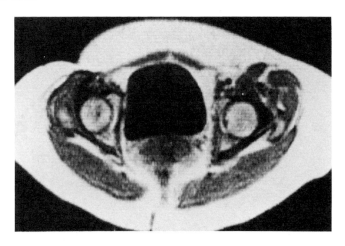

FIG. 10 MR scan showing the blockade of the external iliac artery branch on one side, as indicated by the presence of only one black hole (the vein) on that side.

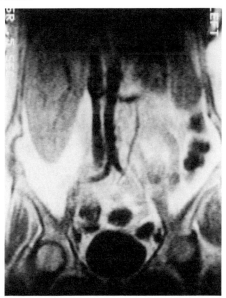

FIG. 11A. MR scan of an aorta with arteriosclerotic plaques.

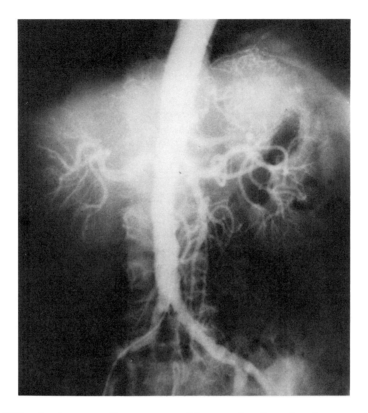

FIG. 11B. Angiogram of an aorta with arteriosclerotic plaques along the lateral wall. Compare with MR scan shown in FIG. 11A on preceding page.

We are now able to progress with MRI detection from larger to smaller abnormalities in spatial terms, but the size of the plaques that can be detected is still too large to have an impact on detection (3,9).

MAGNETIC RESONANCE IMAGING IN CARDIAC DISORDERS

In collaboration with Fletcher et al. (10) we have used MRI to examine pediatric cardiology patients with a variety of lesions. Figure 12 shows a case of tricuspid atresia with thickened tricuspid valve and a small right ventricle. Figure 13 shows a case of atrial septal defect.

In over 50 cases studied thus far, these is an excellent correlation between aortic angrograms and MRI, which has a spatial resolution of about 2 mm.

Figure 14 shows a patient with a penetrating stab wound through the chest, piercing the ventricular septum. Angiogram showed that the contrast medium injected went from the left ventricle through the septum into the right ventricle, confirming this unusual case of artificial ventricular septal defect.

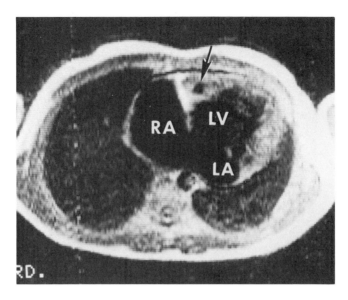

FIG. 12. Axial MR scan at the level of the aortic valve (arrow) in a 7–year old child with an atrial septal defect. RA = right atrium; LA = left atrium; RV = right ventricle. From (10).

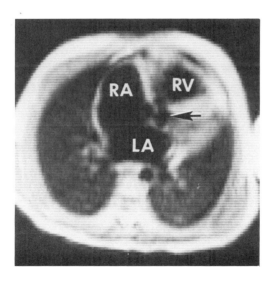

FIG. 13. Axial MR scan of a patient with tricuspid atresia demonstrating thickening wall of the hypoplastic right ventricle (arrow) and an associated atrial septal defect. RA = right atrium; LA = left atrium; LV = left ventricle. From (10).

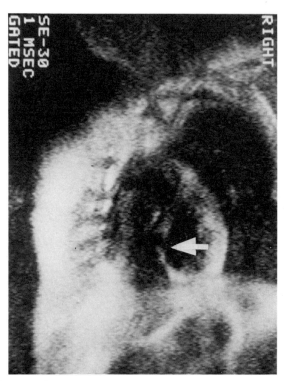

FIG. 14. left anterior oblique MR scan of a patient with a traumatic ventricular septal defect (arrow).

As mentioned above, the key question is whether MRI can be used to detect small infarcts and pre-infarct abnormalities. Gated cardiac MRI was performed on a dog with experimental coronary occlusion induced 2 hr earlier by injecting a pellet into the coronory artery. The imaging showed an infarct in the region of the myocardium corresponding to the area supplied by the occluded vessel. This area correlated well with autoradiographs obtained from myocardial slices containing radioactive microspheres administered into the coronary circulation. Thus, in acutely induced experimental infarcts, we do see a significant change in signal intensity in the myocardium. In a human patient 9 days post-infarct, a similar finding of low signal intensity can be shown on MRI (Figure 15). Figure 16 shows the MRI of an old infarct. These changes correlate well with coronary angiography.

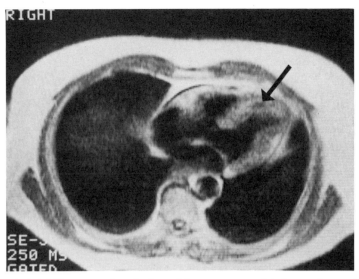

FIG. 15. Axial MR scan of a 9–day old anteroseptal infarct (arrow). ECG cardiac gating. From (5).

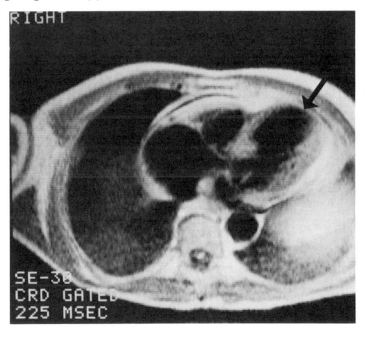

FIG. 16. Axial MR scan of an old anterior wall myocardial infarction (arrow). Note the thin wall. ECG cardiac gating. From (5).

MAGNETIC RESONANCE IMAGING FOR DETECTION
OF EARLY LESIONS

The real paydirt for MRI is the demonstration of vascular lumen narrowing before the occurrence of obstruction and frank infarct. MRI of a post–mortem cast of a carotid artery immersed in a solution containing a paramagnetic substance can show a fairly faithful reproduction of the arterial structure. The problems are (a) the limitation of the spatial resolution (1 mm rather than the 0.5 mm desired), and (b) the picture is only a tomographic slice. Ideally, we would like to obtain 3–D pictures. MRI, like CT, can be reconstructed into 3–D images.

Figure 17A shows a post–mortem cast of human thoracic aorta and coronary vessels. A 3–D MRI image of the distal aorta and proximal coronary branches is shown in Figure 17B. In the intact human patients, one has to deal with respiratory gating and other problems. We would like to reduce significantly the data acquisition time, so that we can see these vessels better. Although we have the ability to identify the coronary artery (Figure 2), it is still not possible to assess whether there is any significant degree of narrowing, because of the insufficient spatial resolution.

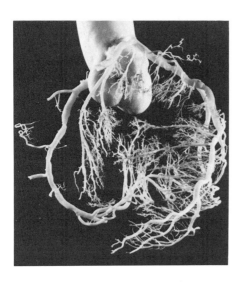
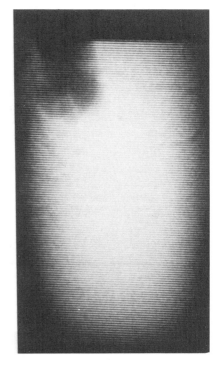

FIG. 17. A (above), B (right),
See legends on next page.

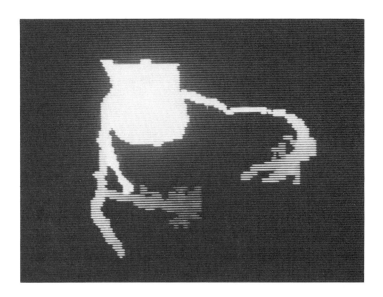

FIG. 17. <u>A</u>, Photograph of a plastic model of the coronary arteries and ascending aorta. <u>B</u>, MR image of the model immersed in a 10^{-4} solution of manganese chloride. The coronary arteries (arrow) appear as a negative signal surrounded by the positive signal from the manganese chloride solution. <u>C</u>, Computer-reconstructed image of the coronary artery model using a surface program. From (5), courtesy of Drs. W. Hinshaw and D. Kramer).

CONCLUSIONS AND PERSPECTIVES

In view of the statistics on the morbidity and mortality on heart attacks and angina, our goals are to improve respiratory gating and spatial resolution, and hopefully to diminish the data acquisition time sufficiently to make it possible to perform limited patient survey techniques. The real question for the future is where do we want to go from here. That is, whether we want to use MR to look at the myocardium per se in terms of capillary flow, or whether we want to look at the coronary arteries. There is also the possibility that we may be able to use hydrogen spectroscopy to see arteriosclerotic plaques and to detect flow. It is to be anticipated that considerable progress will be made in these areas in the near future.

REFERENCES

1. Alfidi, R.J., Haaga, J.R., El Yousef, S.J., Bryan, P.J., Fletcher, B.D., LiPuma, J.P., Morrison, S.C., Kaufman, B., Richey, J.B., Hinshaw, W.S., Kramer, D.M., Yeung, H.N., Cohen, A.M., Butler, H.E., Ament, A.E., and Lieberman, J.M. (1982): Radiology, 143:175–181.
2. Go, R.T., MacIntyre, W.J., Yeung, H.N., Kramer, D.M., Geisinger, M., Chilcote, W., George, C., O'Donnell, J.K., Moodie, D.S., and Meaney, T.F. (1984): Radiology, 150:129–135.
3. Herfkens, R.J., Higgins, C.B., Hricak, H., Lipton, M.J., Crooks, L.E., Sheldon, P.E., and Kaufman, L. (1983): Radiology, 148:161–166.
4. Cheung, N.K., Saarinen, U., Neely, J., Landmeier, B., Donovan, D., and Coccia, P.F. (1985): Cancer Res., 45:2642–2649.
5. Lieberman, J.M., Botti, R.E., and Nelson, A.D. (1984): In: Symposium on Magnetic Resonance Imaging, edited by R.J. Alfidi and J.R. Haaga, pp. 847–858. Radiol. Clin. North Med., vol. 22, W.B. Saunders, Philadelphia.
6. Cohen, A.M. (1984): In: Symposium on Magnetic Resonance Imaging, edited by R.J. Alfidi and J.R. Haaga, pp. 829–846. Radiol. Clin. North Med., vol. 22, W.B. Saunders, Philadelphia.
7. Lanzer, P., Botvinick, E.H., Schiller, N.B., Crooks, L.E., Arakawa, M., Kaufman, L., Davis, P.L., Herfkens, R.J., Lipton, M.J., and Higgins, C.B. (1984): Radiology, 150:121–127.
8. Axel, L., Kressel, H.Y., Thickman, D., Epstein, D., Edelstein, W., Bottomley, P., Redington, R., and Baum, S. (1983): Am. J. Radiol. 141:1157–1162.
9. Lieberman, J.M., Alfidi, R.J., Nelson, A.D., Botti, R.E. Moir, T.W., Haaga, J.R., Kopiwoda, S., Miraldi, F.D., Cohen, A.M., Butler, H.E. et al. (1984): Radiology 152:465–470.
10 Fletcher, B.D., Jacobstein, M.D., Nelson, A.D., Riemenschneider, and Alfidi, R.J. (1984): Radiology 150:137–140.

IV. IN VIVO NMR SPECTROSCOPY

NMR in Biology and Medicine,
edited by Shu Chien and Chien Ho.
Raven Press, New York © 1986.

The Relation Between Muscle Function and Metabolism Studied by ^{31}P NMR Spectroscopy

M. Joan Dawson

Department of Physiology and Biophysics, University of Illinois Medical School at Urbana–Champaign, Urbana, Illinois 61801

When we exercise, the concentration of ATP, the direct fuel for contraction in our active muscles, normally remains unchanged in spite of greatly increased demand. There could be no better demonstration of the tight coupling between cellular function and the metabolic processes which support that function. For over a decade my colleagues and I have been using ^{31}P NMR spectrosocopy to study the relation between mechanical function and metabolism, first in isolated frog muscle and now also in limb muscles of normal human subjects and patients. Our studies and those from other laboratories have led to new and testable hypotheses concerning the control of metabolism and intracellular pH, the nature of fatigue and the mechanism of contraction. This paper will describe some of that work.

MUSCLE BIOCHEMISTRY: AN OVERVIEW

The major biochemical events associated with contraction are summarized in Table I. The sequence of events shown here is well–known and, with differences only in detail, is the basis of energy supply for cellular function in most biological systems. It was first noted by Lipmann in the 1930's that phosphorus–containing compounds play a central role in bioenergetics, a fact which suggests that most bioenergetic systems may be constrained by common thermodynamic and physico–chemical characteristics (cf. 17). In the 1950's it was discovered that the activities of rate–limiting enzymes of glycolysis (reaction sequence 3; Table I) are allosterically affected by phosphorus–containing compounds (see review, 18). Since that time the possibility has been much discussed that these allosteric effectors are responsible for switching metabolic rate up and down in accordance with functional demand.

^{31}P NMR has allowed us an unprecedented opportunity to assess in living tissues present–day theories of metabolic control, which are derived mainly from studies of isolated enzymes. Further, the ability to make measurements that were not possible in the past (e.g. free–energy change for ATP hydrolysis, and relative concentrations of the acid and basic forms of inorganic phosphate, Pi) encourage us to look at the old problems of metabolic control in a new light.

Many of the reactants and allosteric effectors shown in Table I can be observed directly in a ^{31}P NMR spectrum. Others, e.g. ADP, are too low in concentration to be detected, or like lactic acid, do not contain phosphorus. However, enough is known about the biochemistry of skeletal muscle that changes in concentrations of the compounds observed in the ^{31}P spectrum can be used to infer changes in other metabolite concentrations as well. Table II outlines which metabolite concentrations can be determined by ^{31}P NMR, and how this is done in our own and other laboratories. (Further information and justification for the calculations is given elsewhere, e.g. Ref. 9). Depending upon how the experiment is done, the concentrations of all of the initial substrates and final products of each of the pathways shown can either be measured directly or calculated

TABLE I. Major Biochemical Reactions Associated with Contraction [a,b]

Mechanochemical energy conversion:

(1) H_2O + ATP $\xrightarrow[\substack{\text{actomyosin}\\\text{ATPase}}]{}$ ADP + Pi + H^+ ($\Delta G \simeq -60$ kJ mol^{-1})

Anaerobic recovery:

(2) H^+ + PCr + ADP $\underset{\substack{\text{creatine}\\\text{kinase}}}{\xrightleftharpoons{\hspace{1cm}}}$ ATP + Cr ($\Delta G \simeq 0$ kJ mol^{-1})

(3) $1/n(C_6H_{10}O_5)_n$ + 3ADP + 3Pi $\rightarrowtail$ $2(C_3H_5O_3)^-$ + $2H^+$ + $2H_2O$ + 3ATP
$\phantom{(3) 1/n(C_6H_{10}O_5)_n + 3ADP + 3Pi \rightarrowtail 2(C_3H_5}$ lactic acid

Aerobic recovery:

(4) $3O_2$ + 18ADP + 18Pi + $C_3H_6O_3$ $\rightarrowtail$ $3CO_2$ + $20H_2O$ + 18ATP

[a] Details can be found in any comprehensive biochemistry textbook.

[b] Reaction 2 is always near equilibrium and has an equilibrium constant such that (at constant pH) for every 100 molecules of ATP hydrolyzed via reaction one, 99 are re–phosphorylated at the expense of PCr. Reaction sequences 3 and 4 summarize the overall effect of biochemical sequences with several known intermediate steps. Reaction sequence 3 is thought to have a large (exact value in vivo unknown) positive driving force in the direction shown. The activities of rate limiting enzymes are allosterically affected in vitro by phosphorus metabolites, including PCr, ATP, ADP, AMP, IMP and Pi.

indirectly during the course of a ^{31}P NMR experiment. We thus obtain much valuable information concerning concentrations of reactants and allosteric effectors, reaction rates and thermodynamic driving forces.

TABLE II. Methods of Determining Metabolite Concentrations and Other Biochemical Quantities of Interest Using ^{31}P NMR

Direct Observation

1. ATP, PCr (phosphocreatine), Pi (inorganic phosphate): concentrations in units of mmol kg^{-1} wet weight of tissue, determined from spectral peak areas after appropriate calibration.

2. H^+ concentration determined from resonance frequency of Pi on the basis of $H_2PO_4^{1-} \rightleftharpoons H^+ + HPO_4^{2-}$ (pK $\simeq$ 6.8 at 4°C; other ionic species are negligible in living tissues).

Calculations which are valid under equilibrium conditions:

1. [ADP] = [ATP] [Cr] / K [PCr] [H$^+$]

   (creatine kinase equilibrium; K $\simeq$ 2 x 10^9 Mol^{-1})

2. [AMP] = [ADP]^2 / K [ATP]

   (myokinase equilibrium; K $\simeq$ 1.2 Mol^{-1})

Additional calculations valid under some conditions

1.   [Cr]   = Total creatine – [PCr]
   (free creatinine)

2. $[LA^-]$ (lactic acid) $= \dfrac{[\text{prot hist}] [H^+]}{pK_{hist} + [H^+]} + \dfrac{[\text{carnosine}] [H^+]}{pK_{carn} + [H^+]} + \dfrac{[Pi] [H^+]}{pK_{Pi} + [H^+]}$

3. ATP utilization $= 1.5 \Delta[LA^-] - \Delta PCr - \Delta ATP$

4. Free–energy change for ATP hydrolysis

   $\partial G/\partial \xi = \Delta G^{O'} + RT \ln ([ADP][Pi]/[ATP])$

   ($\Delta G^{O'}$ is determined under appropriate conditions of $[H^+]$, $[Mg^{2+}]$)

For full details, see (4,5,6,8,9,22).

Figure 1 shows the results of what is by now a classic type of ^{31}P NMR experiment on muscle contraction and metabolism. In this experiment, isolated frog gastrocnemius muscles were maintained in good physiological condition within a vertical bore high–resolution NMR spectrometer, together with appropriate apparatus for stimulating them electrically and recording their force development. The muscles were exposed to 2 mM NaCN in order to block oxidative phosphorylation (reaction sequence 4, Table I) and to create a closed thermodynamic system in which any metabolite concentration changes are due to chemical reactions and not to movement of substances into or out of the spectrometer sensitive volume. This simplest of possible experiments on whole muscle is directly analogous to intense sprinting–type exercise which results in fatigue before the cardiovascular and respiratory systems can respond with increased oxygen delivery to working muscles.

CAUSES OF MUSCULAR FATIGUE

We search for the underlying biochemical causes of the mechanical changes associated with muscular fatigue, because the knowledge gained is valuable for its own sake, is helpful to the elucidation of the fundamental mechanisms of muscular contraction, and could potentially be useful in devising therapy for muscle diseases that are characterized by abnormal fatigability.

Repetitively stimulated anaerobic muscles quickly display the mechanical manifestations of fatigue, decline in force development and slowing of relaxation that are shown by the inserts in Figure 1. These mechanical changes are accompanied by the metabolic changes shown in the sequentially recorded spectra. There is a gradual loss of PCr, accompanied by an equal build–up of [Pi]. The [ATP], the direct fuel for contraction, remains unchanged as long as there is an adequate supply of PCr (reaction 2, Table I). The gradual shift to the right of the resonance position of the Pi-peak indicates a build–up of lactic acid as ATP is replenished by way of glycogenolysis (reaction 3, Table I).

FORCE FATIGUE

Theories about the cause of force fatigue fall into two broad categories (cf: 3), both of which have substantial experimental support: a) fatigue results from decreased activation of contraction, e.g. a decrease in the amount of Ca^{2+} released from the sarcoplasmic reticulum or its ability to activate the contractile proteins, or b) fatigue results from a decline in the rate of mechanochemical energy conversion by the actomyosin ATPase, as a result of change in concentration of its substrate or products.

In our experiments on fatiguing muscle the pattern of stimulation was altered in such a way that all of the factors associated with the activation of contraction were varied a great deal. We found that the decline in force development was independent of the pattern of stimulation, but as shown in Figures 2A and B was strongly correlated with the build–up of products of ATP–hydrolysis: ADP, Pi and H$^+$. We concluded that force fatigue must result from changes in the concentration of one or more of the products of ATP–hydrolysis, either causing a progressive decline in the activation of contraction or a product–inhibition of actomyosin ATPase activity (8).

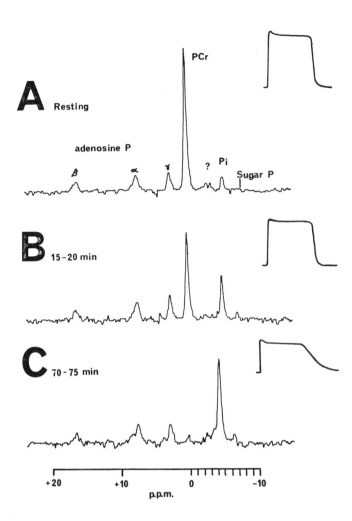

FIG. 1. Spectra and corresponding contractions (inserts) obtained from two anaerobic frog gastrocnemius muscles maintained in physiological salt solution at 4°C within a 7.5 mm diameter NMR sample tube which was converted into an experimental chamber. The muscles were stimulated electrically to maintain a 5 s contraction every 300 s. Spectra were obtained at 129.2 MHz on a spectrometer constructed at the Biochemistry Department, University of Oxford. A: Resting spectrum, obtained after 2 hr anaerobiosis and just before the first stimulation. The first contraction, illustrated by the insert above, showed normal force development and normal mechanical relaxation rate. B and C: The 4th and 16th contractions, respectively. Note the decline in force development and slowing of relaxation association with muscular fatigue. Spectra averaged over sequential 5 min periods showed loss of PCr and building up of Pi (reaction 2, Table I) and acidification as a result of glycogenolysis (reaction 3, Table I). Adapted from (6).

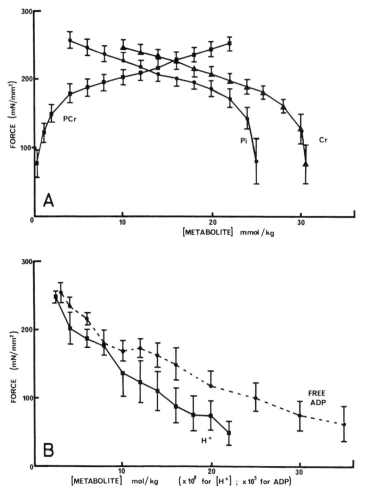

FIG. 2. Force developed as a function of the levels of various metabolites in anaerobic frog gastrocnemius muscles. The results were averaged from 6 experiments (one of which is shown in Fig. 1) in which the muscles were stimulated for 1s/20s, 1s/60s or 5s/300s. Metabolite concentrations were determined from the ^{31}P NMR spectra by the procedures indicated in Table II. From (8).

At the time the experiments shown in Figures 1 and 2 were done, we were unable to say which product or combination of products of ATP hydrolysis might be causally related to mechanical fatigue. Since that time, two pieces of experimental evidence from widely divergent sources have led us to focus primarily on Pi. The first was a ^{31}P NMR study of recovery from contraction in human subjects and the second was a mechanical and biochemical study of single frog muscle fibers from which the cell membrane had been chemically removed.

The NMR study of human subjects was done using a TMR 32 spectrometer system from Oxford instruments (12). The horizontal, 20 cm bore magnet can accommodate limbs of adult human subjects, while a combination of B_0 field profiling and a surface coil allowed selection of approximately 20 cm^3 of forearm grip muscle from which the ^{31}P spectra were obtained. In this study, the subjects were asked to grip a specially designed isometric force transducer as hard as possible (maximum voluntary contraction) for a full three minutes. Spectra were collected before and immediately after the contraction and at 30 s intervals thereafter, until full metabolic and mechanical recovery was attained. The contraction caused large changes in the ^{31}P spectrum which coincided with pronounced mechanical fatigue. Recovery of force development coincided with return of [Pi], but not [H$^+$] or [ADP], toward normal levels (unpublished, Dawson, Edwards, Gordon, Shaw and Wilkie).

Our second reason for relating [Pi] to mechanical fatigue comes from experiments on single skinned frog fibers using "caged ATP" as a method of substrate delivery (10,11). In studies of the relation between changes in metabolite concentrations and mechanical behavior of single fibers, diffusion times are always a limiting factor which complicates interpretation of results. In an attempt to overcome this problem, Goldman and his co-workers bathed the skinned fibers in solutions containing compounds of ATP which are subject to photolysis by bursts of laser light. The muscles were caused to contract (rigor) in various media and subjected to a laser burst. Changes in force development and ATP-hydrolysis rate were noted. In a study in which [ADP] and/or [Pi] in the bathing medium were altered, starting at normal *in vivo* levels in the resting muscle and increasing to levels attained after moderate fatigue, the ATP-hydrolysis rate and force development were markedly affected by changes in [Pi], but not by changes in [ADP] (14).

We therefore had ample reason to focus on the importance of Pi in mechanical fatigue. As noted earlier (see Table II) Pi exists in muscle in two ionic forms, the proportions of which are pH dependent. We have replotted our earlier data obtained from whole frog muscles (Figure 2) to illustrate the relation between force development and ionic species of Pi, as shown in Figure 3. There is a strikingly linear relation between decline in force production and increase in [$H_2PO_4{}^{1-}$]. Since $H_2PO_4{}^{1-}$ is the actual ionic form of the hydrolysis product of ATP, this finding suggests the hypothesis that in normal muscle, force fatigue may be caused by product inhibition of the actomyosin ATPase. Another plausible explanation for this result is that $H_2PO_4{}^{1-}$ may either inhibit Ca-release from the sarcoplasmic reticulum, or efficacy of Ca^{2+} in activating the contractile proteins. Further experiments both on whole muscle and on isolated systems will be necessary in order to distinguish among these possibilities.

RELAXATION FATIGUE

Our ^{31}P NMR studies have also led to a testable hypothesis concerning the mechanism by which the rate of mechanical relaxation changes in fatiguing muscle. A large proportion of the relaxation from an isometric contraction follows a single exponential time course. We found that, like the maximum force achieved, the time constant for the exponential phase

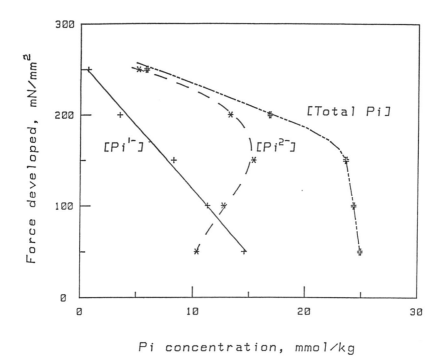

FIG. 3. The relation between force developed and ionic species of Pi. [Total Pi] is re-plotted directly from Figure 2a. [Pi¹⁻] and [Pi²⁻] are the acid and basic forms of Pi, calculated from [Total Pi], [H⁺] and pK = 6.8.

of relaxation ($1/\tau$) was independent of the pattern of contraction, but closely correlated with [ADP], [Pi] and [H⁺]. In all of our experiments there was a tight linear relationship between $1/\tau$ and $dG/d\xi$ for ATP hydrolysis.

This result can be fit into the body of literature on muscle contraction according to the following hypothesis: Mechanical relaxation rate depends not on the time course of actomyosin ATPase activity but upon ATP–dependent re-uptake of Ca^{2+} into the sarcoplasmic reticulum. As muscle fatigues, the rate of Ca^{2+} uptake declines due to a decrease in the free energy change available for this process ($dG/d\xi$ for ATP hydrolysis). Although it may be fortuitous, additional support for the hypothesis comes from a short extrapolation of our results to the X–axis. This shows that relaxation would not occur if $dG/d\xi$ for ATP hydrolysis declined to the value that would be expected to halt Ca^{2+} uptake due to insufficient free energy to drive this process (6).

THE MECHANISM OF MUSCULAR CONTRACTION

One of the fascinating, but still unsolved problems of muscle physiology is the mechanism by which the chemical energy contained within the bond configuration of ATP is converted into mechanical work. Figure 4 shows a scheme for the actomyosin ATPase reaction which conforms to the experimental information available concerning the biochemistry and mechanics of the contraction process. This and other similar schemes can be used to represent the working hypotheses held by most investigators in the field. The form of presentation of Figure 4 was chosen because it can be used to place our ^{31}P NMR results on whole living muscle within the context of information obtained by a variety of other techniques.

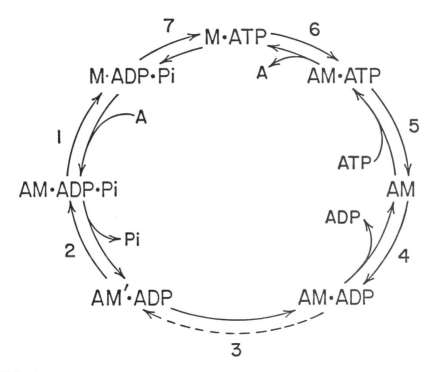

FIG. 4. Proposed biochemical scheme for interaction of actin (A) and myosin (M) to hydrolyze ATP and produce muscular force and movement. This is based largely on the work of Taylor (21) and his associates. Identification of AM'ADP, which can be formed by ATP hydrolysis but not by addition of ADP to AM, is due to Sleep and Hutton (19). Hibberd et al. (14) have shown that reaction 2 is probably reversible and have suggested that formation of the dominant force-generating state is coupled to the release of Pi. The results shown in Figure 3 give strong experimental support for this suggestion and indicate that $H_2PO_4{}^{1-}$ is the actual ionic species of Pi that is involved.

The biochemical cycle of attachment of the contractile proteins, actin and myosin, to one another is powered by the hydrolysis of ATP, as shown in Figure 4, and produces muscular force and movement. The summated effects of numerous independent sites of actomyosin ATPase activity give rise to the mechanical and biochemical behavior of the contracting muscle as a whole. An important characteristic of this cycle is that in resting muscle actin and myosin are largely dissociated and the products of ATP-hydrolysis retained on the myosin. Muscle contraction is initiated by the presence of Ca^{2+} which activates reaction 1, thereby allowing steps 1-4 to proceed in an energetically downhill direction. Evidence has been obtained that reaction 3 is irreversible and that its substrate (AM'ADP) may be the force-generating step (19). As long as ATP and Ca^{2+} continue to be present, the cycle of reactions 1-7 can be continuously repeated.

Increasing Pi is known to reduce force development in skinned fibers (1) and actomyosin ATPase activity in isolated myofibrils. Recently, evidence has been obtained that dissociation of Pi and formation of AM'ADP (reaction 2) may be reversible (14). It therefore follows that physiological changes in Pi could have profound effects on force development and actomyosin ATPase activity. Our ^{31}P NMR results in whole muscle give strong experimental support for this suggestion and indicate that $H_2PO_4^{1-}$ is the actual ionic species of Pi that is involved.

In the steady-state the rate of actomyosin ATPase activity (V) is equal to the forward minus the reverse rate for any of the steps in the cycle. Looking specifically at reaction 2:

$$V = [AM \cdot ADP \cdot Pi] \, k_{for} - [AM' \cdot ADP] \, [Pi] \, k_{rev}$$

Since force production in the whole frog gastrocnemius muscles used in the ^{31}P NMR experiments is proportional to the rate of ATP utilization (8), Figure 3 of this paper indicates that V may be linearly related to the $[H_2PO_4^{1-}]$ product of the actomyosin ATPase cycle. The simplest explanation for this finding is that, during contractions of living muscle, the net rate of reaction 2 determines the rate of actomyosin ATP hydrolysis and therefore the extent of force production. Physiological changes in $[H_2PO_4^{1-}]$ would affect force production by altering the rate of reverse flux through reaction 2.

THE CONTROL OF GLYCOLYSIS

When muscle contracts, the rate of glycolysis increases by several hundred-fold in order to meet the increased demand for ATP. Theories concerning the mechanisms responsible for this increased glycolytic rate generally fall into two broad categories:

(a) Glycolysis might be activated by the same event that triggers contraction itself: Ca^{2+} release from the sarcoplasmic reticulum. In favor of this view, there is evidence that physiological changes in $[Ca^{2+}]$ can, through a series of cascading steps, affect the activity of glycogen phosphorylase, a key rate-limiting enzyme in glycogenolytic sequence (2).

(b) It is widely believed that a negative feedback mechanism exists whereby increases in concentration of direct and indirect products of ATP hydrolysis (see Table II) allosterically activate rate limiting enzymes of glycolysis, thereby increasing the rate of ATP synthesis (see e.g. 20).

Glycolysis Is not Activated by a Metabolic Negative Feedback Mechanism

Our ^{31}P NMR results on frog and human muscle show that a metabolic negative feedback mechanism is not the explanation for increased glyco-lytic rate during contraction and therefore tend to favor hypothesis (a) above.

In repetitively stimulated anaerobic frog gastrocnemii, we have found that glycolysis is activated during each contraction, but quickly comes to a halt despite the fact that phosphorus metabolites have not returned to resting values (Figure 5). Similar results are obtained in humans. The upper panel of Figure 6 shows that when the human forearm is made ischemic for one hour, the [PCr] drops to as low as one half of its initial level with a concomitant rise in [Pi]. Although not shown in Figure 6, it is clear from the equations presented in Table II that [ADP], [AMP] and [IMP] must rise markedly under these conditions. If glycolysis were allosterically activated by increases in the concentrations of these compounds, we would expect a pronounced increase in glycolytic rate. However, as shown by the lower panel of Figure 6, intracellular pH actually goes somewhat <u>alkaline</u> during the ischemic period. This indicates a low glycolytic rate, approximately 3 mmol kg^{-1} hr^{-1} (23).

Figure 7 shows that the situation is dramatically different during a maximal voluntary contraction. In this experiment too, PCr declined by approximately 50 percent, but now the pH fell by a full pH unit, representing a glycolytic rate that is at least 200–fold higher than in the resting ischemic muscle. During the post–contractile ischemic period no metabolic changes could be observed. Similar results have also been obtained in the human quadriceps, using chemical techniques for metabolic analysis (15). We must therefore conclude that whatever activates glycolysis is closely associated with contraction itself (e.g. Ca^{2+} release from the sarcoplasmic reticulum), and not with changes in phosphorus metabolite levels. While the allosteric effects of phosphorus metabolites

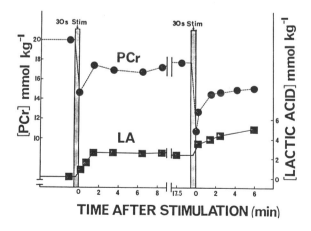

FIG. 5. The time course of changes in [PCr] and [lactic acid] resulting from two 30 s tetani in anaerobic muscles. Note the breaks in the left ordinate and abscissal scales.

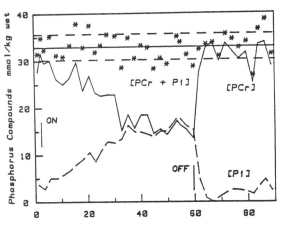

TIME/min (approx 2.5 min bins).

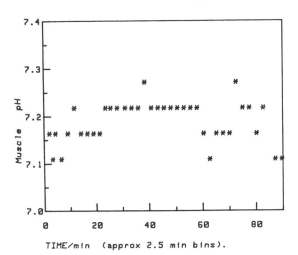

TIME/min (approx 2.5 min bins).

FIG. 6. Upper panel: Changes in [PCr] (solid line) and [Pi] (interrupted line) in forearm muscles during and following 59 min ischemia in the right arm. The sum [PCr+Pi], indicated by *, does not change. An Oxford Research Systems spectrometer with a 20–cm horizontal bore was operated at 32 MHz for ^{31}P. A 4 cm diameter surface coil sampled (80 μs pulses at 2 s intervals) approximately 22 cm^3 of tissue. Details of methods, including conversion of peak areas to absolute concentration, are published elsewhere (23).

Lower panel: Changes in pH during the same experiment as described in the upper panel. The "stepped" changes in pH arise from digitization of resonance frequencies. The pH values observed during the period 20–60 min after onset of ischemia are slightly but significantly more alkaline than the nonischemic values (23).

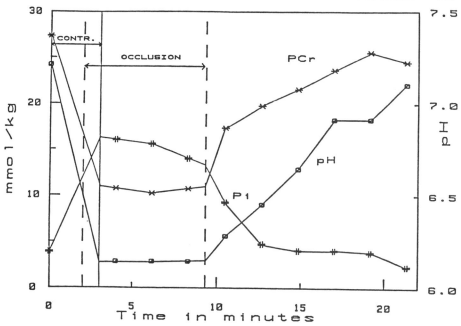

FIG. 7. Changes in PCr, Pi and pH as a result of maximum voluntary isometric contraction. After 2 min of contraction a syphgmomanometer cuff was inflated, contraction was continued for one additional minute, and ischemic conditions were maintained for a further 6 min. Spectra were obtained and calibrated as described for Figure 6.

observed in studies of isolated enzymes of the glycolytic sequence may be of fundamental importance, it is becoming increasingly clear that observation of these effects requires unphysiological concentrations of metabolites (22).

Pi May Have a Fundamental Role In Glycolytic Control

An interesting clue to the mechanism of control of glycolysis in muscle is shown in Figure 8a. Here the final [lactate] produced as a result of any contraction is plotted as a function of the final [PCr] achieved. Figure 8a represents a summary of all of our results in frog muscle obtained at two different temperatures and with widely varying patterns of stimulation. It shows that when a muscle is stimulated to contract, irrespective of the initial [PCr] and regardless of the amount of PCr consumed as a result of the contraction, glycolysis is activated and continues until the relation between [PCr] and [lactate] shown by the curve in Figure 8a is achieved. While this observation is entirely new and perhaps surprising, it does not contradict previously available information. In fact, the literature of the last 50 years on muscle metabolism is full of examples of a constant relation between [PCr] and [lactate], or [PCr] and pH in heavily exercising muscle. So universal a result requires an explanation. (At a minimum it indicates that in the past, conclusions concerning glycolytic rate were erroneously made as a result of experiments in which the <u>extent</u> rather than the <u>rate</u> of glycolysis was the limiting factor).

The explanation for Figure 8a is probably contained in Figure 8b, where [lactate] at the end of an anaerobic recovery period is shown to be proportional to the concomitant $[H_2PO_4^{1-}]$. Earlier in this paper the relation between $[H_2PO_4^{1-}]$ and force development was shown to fit neatly into current literature on the mechanism of muscular contraction and to extend rather than to contradict presently–held theories. The same is not true of our results on the control of glycolysis; the data shown in Figure 8b cannot be easily accommodated by present theories.

Pi enters the glycolytic reaction sequence at only one point (reaction 3, Table I): as a substrate for the rate–limiting enzyme glycogen phosphorylase. The only evidence available indicates that the alkaline form of Pi (HPO_4^{2-}) is the actual species involved (16). Therefore the relation we observe between $H_2PO_4^{1-}$ and the extent of glycolysisis is not explained by a mass action effect of Pi as a reactant. Further, to the best of my knowledge, the allosteric effects of Pi on the various glycolytic enzymes which have been documented in the literature all tend to <u>activate</u> glycogenolysis. Thus, on the basis of mass action or allosteric effects, the apparent inhibition of glycogenolysis by $H_2PO_4^{1-}$ is the opposite of what we would expect.

We are left with two general possibilties: a) there is a previously undescribed inhibitory effect of physiological concentratrations of $H_2PO_4^{1-}$ on the activity of key glycolytic enzymes or b) the observed relation between $H_2PO_4^{1-}$ and extent of glycolysis results from a thermodynamic constraint on this reaction sequence. We have previously suggested (7) that glycolysis might cease when the free–energy change for glycogenolysis declines to a point where it is no longer sufficient to drive the synthesis of ATP. Unfortunately, not enough is know about the thermodynamics of glycogenolysis in living muscle to make a quantitative assessment of this hypothesis.

THE RELATION BETWEEN CONTRACTION AND METABOLISM

One is driven to regard the control of contraction and the control of metabolism as being two interrelated aspects of the same problem. When muscle contracts, metabolic rate increases to meet the greater demand for ATP. However, metabolic processes are not infinite in speed or capacity and therefore mechanical work production must be limited to that which can be supported metabolically. This limitation is most clearly seen under anaerobic conditions, when the rapid onset of mechanical fatigue serves to protect the muscle from ATP depletion and consequent rigor.

A number of metabolites, including ATP and its hydrolysis products, are closely associated with both contraction and metabolism and could therefore function to maintain these two processes in optimum relation to one another. Various substances have been nominated as the critical link, with H+ (13) and Pi (2) receiving the most enthusiasm. The results show in Figures 3 and 8b of this paper give strong quantitative experimental support to the notion that both the contractile process and glycolysis are closely coupled to $[H_2PO_4^{1-}]$ and through this to each other. This suggests a synthesis of the ideas of Hermansen and Chasiotis: the influence of [H+] on contraction and metabolism could well be due to its effect on the proportion of Pi which is present in the form of form of $H_2PO_4^{1-}$.

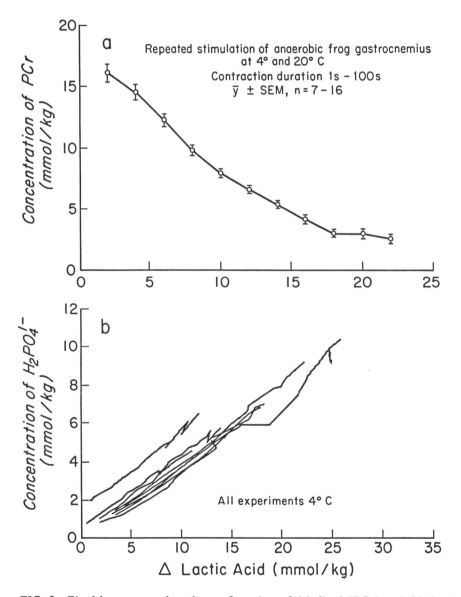

FIG. 8. Final lactate produced as a function of (a) final [PCr] and (b) final [H$_2$PO$_4^{1-}$] achieved after stimulation followed by an aerobic recovery period. For example, data for 17.5 min after the first contraction shown in Figure 5 is represented here. (a) represents a summary of all of our results in frog muscle obtained at two different temperatures and with widely varying patterns of stimulation; (b) represents 7 experiments run at 4°C.

REFERENCES

1. Brandt, P.W., Cox, R.N., Kawai, M., and Robinson, R. (1982): J. Gen. Physiol. 79:997–1016.
2. Chasiotis, D. (1983): Acta Physiological Scandinavica, Suppl. 518:1–68.
3. Ciba Foundation Symposium 82 (1981): Human Muscle Fatigue: Physiological Mechanisms, edited by R. Porter and J. Whelan, Pitman Medical, London.
4. Dawson, M.J. (1982): Bioscience Reports, 2:727–733.
5. Dawson, M.J. (1983): In: Biochemistry of Exercise, edited by H.G. Knuttgen, J.A. Vogel and J. Poortmans, International Series of Sport Science, Vol. 13, pp. 116–125. Human Kinetics Publishers, Champaign, IL..
6. Dawson, M.J., Gadian, D.G., and Wilkie, D.R. (1980): J. Physiol. 299:465–484.
7. Dawson, M.J., Gadian, D.G., and Wilkie, D.R. (1977): NMR in Biology, edited by R.A. Dwek, I.D. Campbell, R.E. Richards, and R.J.P. Williams, pp. 289–321. Academic Press, London.
8. Dawson, M.J., Gadian, D.G., and Wilkie, D.R. (1978): Nature 274:861–866.
9. Dawson, M.J. and Wilkie, D.R. (1984): In: Recent Advances in Physiology, edited by P. Baker, pp. 247–267. Churchill Livingstone, Edinburgh.
10. Goldman, Y., Hibberd, M.G., and Trentham, D.R. (1984): J. Physiol. 354:577–604.
11. Goldman, Y., Hibberd, M.G., and Trentham, D.R. (1984): J. Physiol. 354:604–624.
12. Gordon, R.E., Hanley, P.E., Shaw, D., Gadian, D.G., Radda, G.K., Styles, P., Bore, P.J., and Chan, L. (1980): Nature 287:736–738.
13. Hermansen, L. (1981): In: Human Muscle Fatigue: Physiological Mechanisms, edited by R. Porter and J. Whelan, pp. 75–88. Ciba Foundation Symposium 82.
14. Hibberd, M.G., Dantzig, J.A., Trentham, D.R., and Goldman, Y.E. (1985): Science 228:1317–1319.
15. Hultman, E. and Sjöholm, H. (1983): In: Biochemistry of Exercise, edited by H.G. Knuttgen, J.A. Vogel, and J. Poortmans, pp. 63–75. Human Kinetics Publishers, Champaign, IL.
16. Kasvinsky, P.J. and Meyer, W.L. (1977): Arch. Biochem. Biophys. 181:616–631.
17. Lipmann. F. (1941): Adv. in Enzymology 1:99–162.
18. Rennie, M.J. and Edwards, R.H.T. (1981): In: Carbohydrate Metabolism and Its Disorders, edited by P.J Randle, D.F. Steiner, and W.H. Wheeler, pp. 1–119, Vol. 3. Academic Press, London.
19. Sleep, J.A. and Hutton, R.L. (1978): Biochemistry 17:5423.
20. Stryer, L. (1981): Biochemistry, 2nd edition, W.H. Freeman and Co., San Francisco, CA.
21. Taylor, E.W. (1972): Ann. Rev. Biochem. 41:577–616.
22. Wilkie, D.R. (1983): Biochem. Soc. Trans. 11:244–246.
23. Wilkie, D.R., Dawson, M.J., Edwards, R.H.T., Gordon, R.E., and Shaw, D. (1984): In: Contractile Mechanisms in Muscle: Advances in Experimental Medicine and Biology, edited by H. Pollack and H. Sugi, pp. 333–347, Vol. II.

NMR in Biology and Medicine,
edited by Shu Chien and Chien Ho.
Raven Press, New York © 1986.

Control of Oxidative Metabolism and Hydrogen Delivery in Human Skeletal Muscle. A Steady–State Analysis

J.S. Leigh, Jr., B. Chance, and S. Nioka

*Department of Biochemistry/Biophysics, University of Pennsylvania,
Philadelphia, Pennsylvania 19104*

INTRODUCTION

Whereas analytical biochemistry has great strengths in measuring the more stable components of cell bioenergetics, particularly ATP (as buffered by creatine kinase equilibrium in skeletal tissue, brain and heart [30]), the more labile and indeed interesting components, phosphocreatine (PCr) and inorganic phosphate (P_i) are measured with significantly less accuracy for two reasons. First, the breakdown of PCr during extraction in the interval between cessation of metabolism and assay leads to underestimation of PCr levels and overestimation of P_i. Even more serious is the difficulty in distinguishing, by usual analytical techniques, the bound and free forms and the contents of different intracellular compartments. Thus, ADP, P_i and PCr values obtained by analytical biochemistry may be difficult to quantitatively interpret.

Optical methods have afforded the great advantage of noninvasive measurements of the redox state of electron carriers of the respiratory chain, particularly NADH by fluorometry [15] and cytochromes by spectrophotometry [11]. These redox states are responsive to the substrates; i.e., oxygen and citric acid cycle components, but most important are ADP and P_i and to a lesser extent ATP. Thus, when substrates are in excess, the redox state of the electron carriers, particularly that of NADH, becomes an indicator of the energy state of the tissue as determined by the ADP level localized in the matrix space of the mitochondria. In severe hypoxia, the respiratory chain is regulated by the oxygen concentration instead of the ADP, and NADH and cytochromes become indicators of extremely high sensitivity of the oxygen

---

[1] This is the "complete" version of a paper that has been abbreviated for publication in the Proceedings of the National Academy of Sciences, December 1985.

concentration in the matrix space of the mitochondria. Optical methods are thus paragons of intra-mitochondrial oxygen concentrations. At intermediate concentrations of oxygen, when both ADP and oxygen are controlling, the signals from the electron carriers become difficult to deconvolute. While NADH signals from the body organs require an exposed tissue surface, significant progress has been made in transcranial observation of hemoglobin and cytochrome signals. In both cases, hemoglobin signals interfere and appropriate algorithms for separating redox and oxygen delivery signals are required [13,24,26].

Phosphorus NMR is most sensitive to unbound forms of cell metabolites and affords a wholly noninvasive approach to the study of metabolic control in the cytoplasmic compartment of cells and tissues. ^{31}P NMR can be used to obtain the relative concentrations of PCr, P_i and ATP with rapidity and with significant accuracy ($\pm$ 10 percent in one minute). These concentration ratios are of great usefulness and importance in the study of metabolic control in animal models, neonates, and adults. Additional information is available when the absolute values of tissue concentrations of PCr and P_i are calculated from the value of ATP, and also creatine, as determined by analytical biochemistry (or prospectively by proton NMR [2,3]). When ADP plays its usual role as a regulatory metabolite, its concentration is maintained at a level too low to be determined by NMR and instead can be calculated directly from the PCr/P_i value with appropriate assumptions. Under these conditions, NMR becomes a very useful tool because the principal elements of energy metabolism are determined and thermodynamic values may be calculated. As we shall discuss here, velocities of oxidative metabolism relative to their maxima for the particular tissue conditions may be determined with significant accuracy in the region of cell pH's between 7.4 and 6.8 and with appropriate corrections below 6.8. We shall show how P-NMR can be used, particularly in tissues stressed with hypoxia, for the prediction of stability, quasi-stability, and instability of oxidative metabolism in relation to the particular workload or functional ATPase activity.

Explanations of the response of body organs to ischemia and hypoxia have been offered from time to time [37] and most of them suggest that the primary event on the pathway to cell damage involves an acidosis. The effects may be catastrophic upon the functionality of both oxidative and glycolytic phosphorylation and upon ionic equilibria. A key question arises, namely, is there an intrinsic property of oxidative metabolism in a hypoxic/ischemic stressed tissue which renders it susceptible to a metabolic catastrophy with minimal acidosis and which may be exacerbated by greater acidosis. We term such a possibility a "kinetic failure" as opposed to an "acidotic failure". The kinetic failure occurs when the ATP synthesis by mitochondria fails to meet the needs of the functional ATPase and a steady state can no longer be maintained, and a "metabolic brain death occurs" [31,36]. Thus the instability of oxidative metabolism can be caused by its incapability for adequate metabolic work, which as we describe below, can be evaluated by the PCr/P_i ratio.

METABOLIC CONTROL

Control of oxidative metabolism includes not only the delivery of ADP and P_i from the functional ATPases, but also of oxygen from the capillary circulation and the delivery of substrates to form NADH as indicated by the equation where the value of 3.0 is appropriate [32]:

$$3ADP + 3P_i + NADH + H^+ + 1/2\ O_2 = 3\ ATP + NAD^+ + H_2O \quad (1)$$

A choice between ADP, P_i, and ATP, as control chemicals for the rate of Eq. (1) is equal insofar as the equations below are concerned, but P–NMR has permitted a much more precise evaluation of this often vexing question [6]. Under various conditions, all of the substrates and products (except H_2O) might possibly serve as control chemicals. The control of respiration by ADP was first characterized by Chance and Williams [12], however, biochemical assays of extracted tissues from various sources consistently reveal high ADP levels that change only by small fractions of the tissue metabolic rates.

Metabolic control by inorganic phosphate was favored by both Racker [41] and Lynen [33], because analytical biochemistry showed large metabolism–linked variations of P_i levels in yeast cells [10]. Recently, phosphorus NMR studies in vivo have begun to explain this old problem. Quantitative measurements in vitro showed the K_m for control of respiration in isolated mitochondria by P_i to be about 1 mM. NMR studies of human skeletal muscles show the resting (state 4) values of P_i to be in the range of 1 to 4 mM. By way of contrast, the values of ADP concentrations calculated from the P–NMR data in the resting state are < 10 μM, well below the K_m, consistent with ADP control of the respiration rate. In functional activity, in the transition from resting state 4 to the active state 3, the functional ATPase produces equal amounts of ADP and P_i. Due to the hundred–fold ratio of P_i/ADP, ADP levels rise 100 times more rapidly in proportion than does P_i, thus ensuring what amounts to ADP control of the resting state 4 to the active state 3 transition.

Metabolic control by NADH–generating substrates is possible; for example, in insulin–induced glucose deficiency [4], the maximal capacity of ATP synthesis will decline. Under such conditions, the redox state of NADH shows oxidation well beyond that characteristic of the controlled state 4 or even the active state 3, a distinctive signal of deficiency of reducing substrate [12].

Analytical biochemistry gives indirect support to the idea of P_i control, since ADP concentrations based on the analysis of total cell content give values that are many fold the K_m [ADP] in resting muscle [12]. However, it is well known that a large fraction of the total cellular ADP is bound to various protein sites and thus unavailable for oxidative phosphorylation. This "bound" ADP is composed of two different classes of binding sites. Those ADP sites exchange with the pool of free ADP at a much slower rate than metabolic pool turnover times, i.e. longer than 1 min. This type of bound ADP is exemplified by the "structurally bound" ADP in actin and GDP in tubulin filaments. In skeletal muscle, heart and brain, this form may abount to 240, 160, and 320 n moles/gm tissue [34,38,39,40].

Other forms of "bound ADP" include that which is bound at enzyme active sites, e.g., creatine kinase, myosin, etc. While this form of ADP is in rapid equilibrium with the unbound pool, the equilibrium ratios of bound ATP/ADP are commonly near unity [35] and thus highly distorted from normal steady state values for the unbound pools. Substantial portions of non–cytoplasmic ADP are also identified with intra–organellar fractions. The intramitochondrial pool in heart and red skeletal muscle is particularly large due to the very high mitochondrial content. Bound ADP at allosteric control sites on various enzymes also accounts for a small fraction of the cellular ADP. The difficulties involved with properly delineating the various forms of metabolically active and non–metabolically active ADP by biochemical extraction techniques are overwhelming, but rarely fully appreciated. It is probably fair to say that this accounting has never yet been accomplished at a precision necessary for quantitative bioenergetic assessment.

Studies of isolated mitochondria showed that serial additions of increasing concentration of ADP resulted in a "Michaelis–Menten response" of respiratory activity with a half maximal value of about 20 µM [12]. At the same time, it was found that NADH showed a half maximal oxidative response between the resting ADP deficient state 4 and fully activated, ADP saturated state 3 [8]. By using the NADH response to ADP, as observed in vitro as an in vivo ADP indicator in stimulated muscles, both perfused and in situ, a similar sensitivity of mitochondria in vivo to ADP produced in single twitches was demonstated [7,8,16]. These early observations identified free ADP in the cytosol as sensed by the mitochondrial translocase to be in the range of the K_m, only a small fraction of the bound plus free forms of ADP as measured by analytical biochemistry and consistent with that estimated by NADH fluorometry of the tissues. P–NMR results are especially relevant here since the freely tumbling form is measured and found to be much below the total ADP as measured by analytical biochemistry and consistent with that estimated by NADH fluorometry. Similar discrepancies are found in brain [21].

A MODEL

A steady state model simulates the physiological condition crucial to life [5]. In Figure 1, ATP synthesis must match ATP breakdown in a feedback control loop. Activation of the functional ATPase to break down ATP produces ADP and phosphate which is translocated into the mitochondrial matrix to activate oxidative phosphorylation. The key feature of the system is that the ADP and phosphate concentrations regulate the rate of oxidative phosphorylation exactly to meet the needs of the functional ATPase so a homeostasis of the ATP level is obtained from this stable feedback loop. At the same time, the level of ATP is temporally and spatially buffered by the creatine kinase equilibrium, so that sudden changes of functional ATPase activity cannot cause wide swings of the rate of oxidative phosphorylation. As the levels of ADP and phosphate rise, glycolytic activity is similarly increased. As ATPase rates approach the maximal rate of oxidative phosphorylation, glycolysis takes over an increasing proportion of the metabolic burden. Thus, for each level of functional activity, there will be particular concentrations of the control chemical, ADP.

The transfer function relates velocities or tissue work rates to the concentration of the control chemicals. There can be a transfer function for ADP, P_i, oxygen, substrate, or any of the parameters of Eq. (1) above. The intersection of the work or load line with the transfer function is termed the operating point. The operating point is confined to move along the transfer function as the work varies. We determine the transfer function in vivo by an arm exercise protocol.

DERIVATION OF MICHAELIS–MENTEN RELATIONSHIP
IN TERMS OF NMR PARAMETERS

NMR perceives only indirectly the concentration of a control chemical such as ADP through the creatine kinase equilibrium and measures directly two major components of this equilibrium, namely, ATP and phosphocreatine (PCr).

A suitable transfer function for metabolite control of oxidative phosphorylation is the simple Michaelis–Menten expression:

$$\frac{V}{V_{max}} = \frac{1}{1 + (K_m/[ADP])} \tag{2}$$

The K_m for ADP control in the presence of saturating P_i and with negligible ATP was initially determined to be 20 μM [12,27]. This relationship varies somewhat with pH in a bell shaped curve symmetrical about the physiological pH [9]. Use of this simple form neglects the effects of the other substrate P_i and the product ATP. Thus, one may not expect complete agreement with experimental results. The NMR parameters can conveniently be entered into this equation from the creatine kinase equilibrium.

$$PCr + ADP + H^+ \xrightarrow{K} ATP + Cr \tag{3}$$

$$[ADP] = \frac{[Cr] \times [ATP]}{[PCr] \times [H^+]} \tag{4}$$

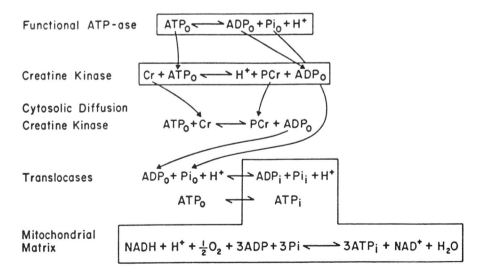

FIG. 1. Illustrating the feedback interactions of the cytosolic and mitochondrial compartments of the muscle cell.

For this discussion, we shall assume a constant pH of 7.1, a temperature of 37°C, a 1 mM free magnesium concentration and a 5 mM ATP concentration, giving $K_1 \times [H^+] = 130\ (30)$, $K_m\ ADP = 2 \times 10^{-5}\ M$ (12):

Substituting these parameters into Eq. (2), we obtain

$$\frac{V}{V_{max}} = \frac{1}{1 + \dfrac{0.52}{[Cr]/[PCr]}} \tag{5}$$

However, it is useful for P–NMR spectroscopy to measure the ratio of PCr/P_i, since this compensates for scale factor and other changes. Under our conditions of steady state exercise, we observe $PCr+P_i$ to be constant to approximately ± 10% [14]. Analytical data show that $PCr+Cr$ is constant in a variety of studies. Sensitive proton NMR can eventually afford the sum of PCr and Cr as well as the ratio. Since the increments of Cr and P_i are necessarily equal in exercise over a range of 2 to 12 mM, relatively small inequalities of Cr and P_i are negligible at higher work loads and large P_i values. Replacement of Cr with P_i leads to the approximate expression:

$$\frac{V}{V_{max}} = \frac{1}{1 + \dfrac{0.52}{[P_i]/[PCr]}} \tag{6}$$

CONTROL BY ADP+P_i

The possibility that both ADP and P_i contribute to in vivo metabolic control is suggested by our observation in isolated mitochondria that the reduction of NAD by succinate required ATP:

$$\text{succinate} + ATP + NAD^+ \rightarrow \text{fumarate} + NADH + ADP + P_i + H^+ \tag{7}$$

It was further found that reduced cytochrome c was oxidized in anaerobic mitochondria by addition of ADP and that an $ATP/(ADP \times P_i)$ ratio of $10^4\ M^{-1}$ characterized the half–potential of this reaction. These results were confirmed and extended by Klingenberg [28], whose results suggested that respiration was governed by an $ATP/(ADP \times P_i)$ ratio of $1.6 \times 10^4\ M^{-1}$. Thus it is important to recognize whether or not these results are of importance in exercised muscle as studied here.

A modification of Eq. (2) to this point gives:

$$\frac{V}{V_{max}} = \frac{1}{1 + \dfrac{ATP \times 6.3 \times 10^{-5}}{P_i \times ADP}} \tag{8}$$

Substitution of the creatine kinase equilibrium then yields:

$$\frac{V}{V_{max}} = \frac{1}{1 + \dfrac{8.1 \times 10^{-3}/Cr}{P_i/PCr}} \qquad (9)$$

For creatine concentration of 15 mM, this formulation predicts a P_i/PCr "K_m" of 0.54.

Thus, the transfer function between work, V/V_{max}, and the biochemical response, P_i/PCr, is expected to approximate a rectangular hyperbola with "K_m" $\simeq 0.5$ to 1. We have therefore explored this relation in detail over the past several years [14,25] in order to determine how well this simple equation fits the muscle exercise data and if so, what the experimental value of K_m' may be.

STEADY STATE EXERCISE PROTOCOL

Since the above relations apply to the steady state with pH and oxygen delivery being constant, the subject is asked to perform graded levels of exercise, in a steady state protocol from rest to approximately K_m; i.e., $P_i/PCr \leq 1.0$. The work is quantitatively evaluated by an ergometer coupled to the exercised limb, and the P_i/PCr value is measured by a surface coil placed upon the exercising muscle. Thus this is an essential "aerobic exercise" and contrasts with other exercise protocols that are carried out to the point of "fatigue", lactic acidosis, etc. and generally non–steady state conditions [1]. Occasionally, we increase the work to near V_{max} to identify the maximal work capability, but do not normally include this as part of the transfer function analysis.

Figure 2 illustrates a typical protocol for evaluation of steady state [14], endurance performance through the work vs. P_i/PCr relationship. Each 5 min measurement interval is preceded by an interval of 3 min to ensure that a steady state is achieved that declines less than 10 percent during the 5 min measurement interval. This protocol also affords a "maximal bout" at the end of the steady state interval in order to validate the V_{max} calculation.

EXPERIMENTAL RESULTS

Figure 3 shows a typical transfer characteristic for an endurance performance test of a human arm where the work is varied from 10 to 35 J/min and the corresponding values of P_i/PCr increase from the rest value of 0.1 to a value slightly over 1. The form of the curve in this case approximates a rectangular hyperbola. The experimental data are well fit to Eq. (6) with a V_{max} of 59 J/min and a K_m of 0.65 ± 0.06. This corresponds to K_m ADP = 25 μM. We can also use these values to calculate that the resting state value of V/V_{max} is approximately 0.1.

The transfer function is also well fit by Eq. (9) with a V_{max} of 48.7 J/min, assuming a total creatine (Cr + PCr) concentration of 30 mM, and Cr = P_i + 10 mM. This yields a "K_m" $\simeq 0.50$.

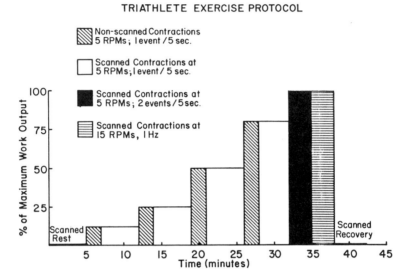

FIG. 2.   Illustrating the steady state graded protocols of the human limb showing rest and contraction intervals.   Each interval of measured performance preceded by a warmup interval.

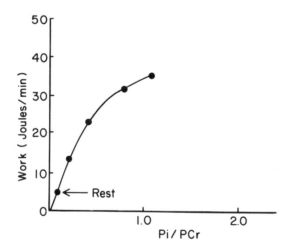

FIG. 3.   A graded exercise response transfer function for an individual with vasomotor response exceeding the tissue of oxygen demand.   A Michaelis–Menten rectangular hyperbola fits the data to ±10% for the parameters exhibited in the figure. The value of K_m' is converted to K_m ADP of 28 ± 3 μM, as compared with 20 μM observed by Chance and Williams (12).

EFFECT OF REGULATION OF OXYGEN DELIVERY ON
THE TRANSFER FUNCTION

Figure 4 represents a protocol obtained from the work $\underline{vs}$. P_i/PCr curve for an Olympic aspirant in an early stage of training. The observed transfer function is not a good fit to a rectangular hyperbola.

One explanation of the difference between the transfer characteristics of Figures 3 and 4 is that oxygen delivery in an athletically trained muscle is adjusted to meet the tissue needs up to the inflection point of the curve. The adjustment of O_2 delivery is regulated by a negative feedback or homeostatic control that minimizes the fluctuations of the ADP or P_i/PCr levels. The transfer characteristic is therefore steeper or "stiffened" as P_i/PCr increases with increasing work.

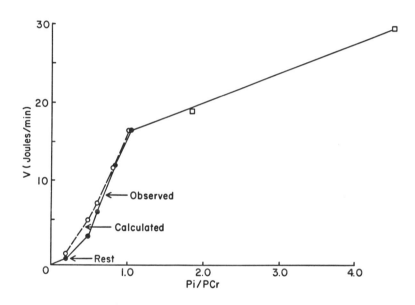

FIG. 4. The transfer function for an individual who has not experienced vasodilation prior to the arm exercise test. The characteristic is steeper and exhibits a sharp break point. This transfer characteristic is attributed to a combination of increased oxygen delivery to oxygen–limited tissue volumes together with the Michaelis–Menten hyperbolic transfer characteristic for ADP control. The increase of V_{max} is indicated here to be proportional to P_i/PCr. The calculated value of V_{max} shown here by the solid circles increases slightly more rapidly than the transfer characteristic itself, suggesting that oxygen delivery "keeps ahead" of the exercise performance need. The increase of V_{max} is over a factor of 2 in the exercise performance.

If one assumes that oxygen delivery to tissue is proportional to the ADP or P_i/PCr value of the tissue and that V_{max} varies approximately as $k\,P_i/PCr$, substitution in Eq. (6) above gives

$$V = \frac{k\,P_i/PCr}{1 + \dfrac{0.52}{[P_i]/[PCr]}} \qquad (10)$$

For values of P_i/PCr greater than $K_m{'}$, the transfer function is a straight line of slope k, whilst for values of P_i/PCr less than K_m, the curve is quadratic and joins the rest value of P_i/PCr. We have calculated the values V for the five points on the early portion of the transfer function for K = 22 Joules/min (open circles), which is seen to yield a fairly good approximation to the data.

In this transfer characteristic, ADP or P_i/PCr regulation of oxidative metabolism is complemented by regulation of oxygen delivery to give a tighter feedback control and a more precise homeostasis which minimizes the variation of P_i/PCr. At high P_i/PCr, glycolytic phosphorylation becomes increasingly activated and supplements mitochondrial oxidative phosphorylation.

TRANSFER CHARACTERISTICS OF THE HEART

The heart can be considered to be the organ of the body which is maximally adapted to endurance performance, in fact for the lifetime of individual. This may be especially true in the cardiac performance of "pursuit" type of animals such as dogs, compared with "sprint" type of animals such as cats. We have therefore selected the beagle dog as an example of an endurance performer and have made preliminary P NMR measurements of the transfer function of the cardiac tissue (Fig. 5). The NMR surface coil is implanted via a left thorocotomy and is glued directly to the surface of the left ventricle [20,29]. While the accurate measurement of heart work is difficult, we have employed the rate pressure product as an approximation. Stimulation by various levels of work by isoproterenol have been used. The values of P_i include a substantial component due to the blood 2,3–diphosphoglycerate as seen through the approximately 1 cm ventricular wall by the 1.5 cm diameter surface coil. The transfer characteristic is nearly linear, consistent with an increase of V_{max} with workload according to Eq. (10). Here the set point for regulation is at a PCr/P_i value of approximately 10 or about one sixth of V_{max}. This extremely conservative operating point permits increases of V without reaching saturation of oxygen delivery and oxidative metabolism. This high value of phosphate potential may be required for endurance performance, so that maximal functional activity does not lead to lactic acidosis.

Preliminary experiments on new born lambs and cats suggest that the transfer functions differ from that observed in Figure 5, presumably because of lack of maturation or lack of need for endurance performance in the cat [20].

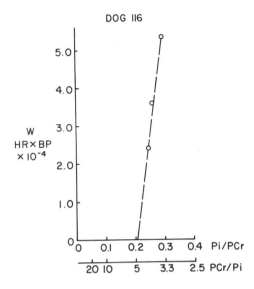

FIG. 5. Work–P_i/PCr transfer function for the heart of an anesthetized beagle dog obtained from a surface coil implanted on the cardiac tissue. The work as varied by increasing i.v. levels of isoproterenol is approximated by the rate pressure product and P_i/PCr is measured directly from the spectra on the assumption that 2,3–DPG makes a constant contribution. The steep slope suggests an even more efficient autoregulation in response to oxygen demand than in the human arm exercise protocol.

PERTURBATIONS: OXYGEN AND pH

Perturbations imposed upon the ADP transfer characteristics are simply expressed in graphical form, where V_{max} for the ADP control characteristic is modulated by one or more parameters: in this case, the tissue oxygen concentration. The oxygen control characteristic is also hyperbolic as determined experimentally [17]. The value of the Michaelis–Menten affinity for oxygen control is given by the expression $K_m O_2 = k_3/k_1$, where k_3 is the turnover number (5 sec^{-1} in state 4 to 50 sec^{-1} in state 3) and k_1 is the second order velocity constant for the reaction of cytochrome oxidase with oxygen (5×10^7 M^{-1} sec^{-1}) [18]. Thus, if we take an activity, double the rest level ($\simeq$ 10/sec), the K_m is 2×10^{-7} M or 0.1 torr. This transfer function is displayed on the right hand side of Figure 6. The oxygen concentration (0.15 torr) available to the mitochondria is slightly above K_m, the corresponding V_{max} for oxygen utilization sets the asymptote of the transfer characteristic for ADP control (left portion of the graph). For a given workload, A_w, the operating point as defined above is at point A_3 giving values of ADP and

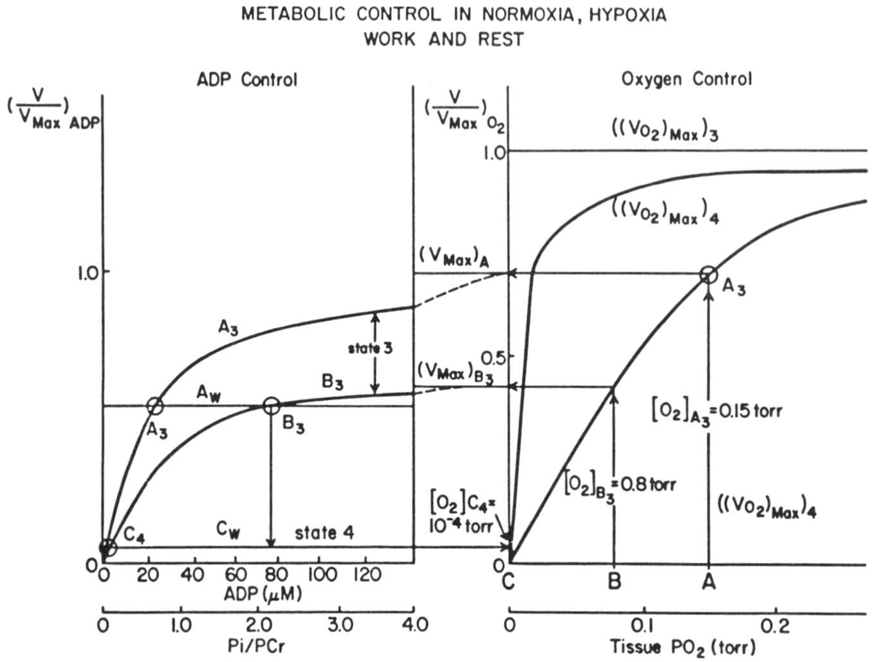

FIG. 6. A calculated transfer function on Michaelis–Menten mechanisms for oxygen control (right), and ADP control (left) at constant pH and variable oxygen delivery and work load. Note that a small change of oxygen delivery (A → B) causes a large change of P_i/PCr (A_3 → B_3) and that decreasing work load causes a large decrease of the oxygen requirement (B → C).

P_i/PCr of 25 µM and 0.66, respectively. Under these conditions, the system is stable and well controlled. Fluctuations in the oxygen delivery to tissue will move the operating point for oxygen delivery along the rectangular hyperbola, resulting in a different V_{max} for the ADP transfer function; for example, there is a 50% decrease of the oxygen concentration from point A to point B, the maximum of the ADP transfer function will be lowered proportionally, giving the transfer characteristics of B_3. The operating point now moves from P_i/PCr of 1.5 to 2.2, and ADP from 25 to 77 µM.

Unstable or Poorly Controlled Metabolic States

The operating point is now at a quasi–stable or poorly uncontrolled point, since further diminutions of the oxygen delivery moves point B_3 to the left in the oxygen control diagram and to the right in the ADP control diagram.

It is apparent that the unstable or poorly controlled operating point involves a great deal of positive feedback, namely, the high ADP concentrations activate glycolysis and cause a lactic acidosis, which will further deteriorate the ADP control transfer function by inhibiting oxidative phosphorylation [9]. Possible therapeutic procedures are: i) to restore the oxygen concentration; ii) to decrease the workload (as in skeletal tissues); and iii) to correct the acidity. In organs such as brain and heart, cessation of function is self–defeating for the heart or not possible for the brain. Thus if the brain ATPase rate exceeds the ATP synthesis rate, a metabolic brain death readily occurs as the operating point moves to higher and higher ADP and P_i/PCr concentrations and no steady state is possible. Furthermore, the metabolic load line is likely to rise due to the high extracellular potassium concentrations causing maximal rate of the transport ATPase. Similarly, with the heart, hypoxia may cause a tachycardia, raising the load line of an already stressed cardiac tissue. In this case, cardiac arrest will cause ischemia and lower the tissue PO_2 drastically.

Perturbation by pH

The creatine kinase equilibrium is pH sensitive and, as indicated in Eq. (5), the "K_m" increases linearly with $[H^+]$, showing that the P_i/PCr value must rise to maintain V/V_{max} constant in acidosis. This has been verified in muscle exercise in hypercapnia where the P_i/PCr increase has matched the H^+ increase, with a 10 to 20 percent decrease of V_{max}.

Heterogeneity of Oxygen Delivery

A diagram similar to that of Figure 6 illustrates how the heterogeneity of oxygen delivery can cause a portion of the tissue volume under observation to be in a quasi–stable or poorly controlled state, whilst the remainder of the tissue volume is in a stable state. The right hand portion of Figure 7 illustrates the oxygen control characteristics similar to those of Figure 6. The dashed curve shows a distribution of oxygen concentrations similar in shape to that observed by Kessler using the oxygen microelectrode [23]. At point A, the oxygen concentration is adequate to maintain operating point at P_i/PCr $\simeq$ 0.6 and ADP $\simeq$ 20 μM [12]. If, however, the tissue volume under observation has oxygen concentrations denoted by C and below, the operating point now moves to point C, with P_i/PCr > 2 and ADP > 70 μM. Further, tissue volumes at the low PO_2 limb of the oxygen distribution profile afford V_{max}'s which are tangent to the load line or significantly below it. This volume of the tissue is in an unstable state, while the bulk of tissue volume is in a well controlled state. Obviously, changing patterns of oxygen delivery [19] can shift tissue volume in a poorly controlled state so that accumulation of damage may not occur.

The sharp border zones observed experimentally in model coronary artery occlusion lead to an abrupt change of the NADH redox state in a distance of 100 microns on the surface of the heart as determined by redox scanning or by microanalysis [22]. Thus, the sharpness of the border zone between normoxic and hypoxic tissues depends on both steep oxygen gradients and the nature of the instability of metabolic control when the

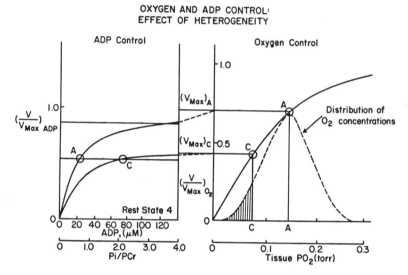

FIG. 7. Illustrating the effect of a distribution of oxygen concentrations upon the metabolic operating point: A, tightly controlled and stable; C, poorly controlled and unstable. Tissue volumes to the left of C are poorly controlled and quite unstable.

operating point is in region C. The unstable response of P_i/PCr and ADP at point C and below is mirrored in the abrupt transition of the redox state of NADH, for example, as the work load is increased towards V_{max} [4]. Thus the simple graphical analysis affords explanations of many of the metabolic control phenomena that have been only dimly perceived in the past.

SUMMARY

This article describes the thermodynamic and kinetic significance of P–NMR spectroscopy for in vivo detection of energy related compounds: PCr, P_i and ATP. The ratio of PCr/P_i is closely related to the phosphate potential of the particular organ under study. The idea of transfer function (work output vs. biochemical input) is developed for various organs of the body under steady state conditions. For metabolic control by the ADP concentration, the work load of each organ identifies an operating point on an approximately hyperbolic transfer function characterized by an ADP concentration and a corresponding P_i/PCr value as seen by P–NMR. Based upon Michaelis–Menten kinetics and the in vitro parameters in the creatine kinase equilibrium, we find that a K_m of 25 μM ADP (corresponding to P_i/PCr of 0.65 ± 0.06) fits the data from an experimental exercise protocol performed by a particular well–trained athlete, whose transfer function is characterized by a rectangular hyperbola. Circulatory control of oxygen delivery to an oxygen–limited organ may alter the transfer function to a sigmoidal curve which is fitted by V_{max} proportional to the ADP (or P_i/PCr level). The transfer function for the heart of an endurance performance animal (dog) shows highly effective regulation. The effects of pH are readily explained, as are those of microheterogeneity. The experimental data and theoretical derivations indicate that a single measurement of P_i/PCr by P-NMR justifies a calculation of the fraction of maximal activity (V/V_{max}) at which a particular organ is operating in the steady state. This quantity appears to be useful in diagnosis and therapy of metabolic disease in the organs of neonates and adults.

ACKNOWLEDGMENTS

This work was supported by NIH Grants HL 31934, HR 34004, RR 02305 and AA 05662, and by the Benjamin Franklin Partnership's Advanced Technology Center of Southeastern Pennsylvania.

REFERENCES

1. Arnold, D.L., Matthews, P.M., and Radda, G.K. (1984): Mag. Reson. in Med. 1:307–315.
2. Arus, C., Barney, M., Westler, W.M., and Markley, J.L. (1984): J. Mag. Res. 57:519–525.
3. Behar, K.L., den Hollander, J.A., Stromski, M.E., Ogini, T., Shulman, R.G., Petroff, O.A., and Prichard, J.W. (1983): Proc. Natl. Acad. Sci. 80:4945–4948.
4. Behar, K.L., den Hollander, J.A., Petroff, O.A.C., Hetherington, H.P., Prichard, J.W., and Shulman, R.G. (1985): J. Neurochem. 44:1045–1055.
5. Burton, A. (1939): J. Cell. Comp. Physiol. 14:327–349.
6. Chance, B. (1959): In: Regulation of Cell Metabolism, edited by C.E.W. Wolstenholme, and C.M. O'Conner, pp. 91–121. J. and Churchill, Ltd., London.
7. Chance, B. (1959): N.Y. Acad. Sci. 81:477–489.
8. Chance, B. (1965): J. Gen. Physiol. 49:163–188.
9. Chance, B. and Conrad, H. (1959): J. Biol. Chem. 234:1568–1570.
10. Chance, B. and Hess. B. (1955): Ann. New York Acad. Sci. 63:1008–1016.
11. Chance, B. and Jobsis, F. (1959): Nature 184:195–196.
12. Chance, B. and Williams, G. (1955): J. Biol. Chem. 217:383–393.
13. Chance, B., Barlow, C., Nakase, Y., Takeda, H., Mayevsky, A., Fischetti, R., Graham, N., and Sorge, J. (1978): Am. J. Physiol. 235:H809–820.
14. Chance, B., Eleff, S., Sokolow, D., and Sapega, A. (1981): Proc. Natl. Acad. Sci. 78:6714–6718.
15. Chance, B., Graham, N., and Mayer, D. (1971): Rev. Sci. Instr. 42:951–957.
16. Chance, B., Mauriello, G., and Aubert, X.M. (1962): In: Muscle as a Tissue, edited by K. Rodahl and S.M. Horvath, pp. 128–145. McGraw-Hill, New York.

17. Chance, B., Oshino, N., Sugano, T., and Mayevsky, A. (1973): In: <u>Oxygen Transport to Tissues</u>, edited by H. Bicher and D. Burley, pp. 239–244.Plenum Publ. Co., New York.
18. Chance, B., Schoener, B., and Schindler, F. (1964): In: <u>Oxygen in the Animal Organism</u>, edited by F. Dickens and E. Neil, pp. 367–388. Pergamon Press, London.
19. Chang, B.L., Yamakawa, T., Nuccio, J., Pace, R., and Bing, R.J. (1984): <u>Circulation Res</u>. 50:240–249.
20. Clark, B.J., Hilberman, M., Subramanian, H., Nioka, S., Schnall, M., Holland, G., Egan, J. Osbakken, M., Chance, B., and Rashkind, W.J. (1985): <u>Ped. Res</u>. 19:125.
21. Granholm, L. and Siesjo, B.K. (1969): <u>Acta Physiol. Scand</u>. 75:257–266.
22. Harken, A.H., Barlow, C.H., Harden, III, W.R., and Chance, B. (1978): <u>Am. J. Cardiol</u>. 42:954–959.
23. Hauss, J., Schonleben, K., Spiegel, V., and Kessler, M. (1978): In: <u>Oxygen Transport to Tissue–III</u>, edited by I. Silver, M. Erecinska, and H. Bicher, pp. 419–422. Plenum Press, New York.
24. Jobsis, F.F. (1985): <u>Adv. & Exp. Med. & Biol</u>. In press.
25. Kent, J., Chance, B., Leigh, J.S., Jr., Maris, J., O'Toole, M., and Hiller, D. (1985): <u>Fed. Proc</u>. 44:1371.
26. Kimura, S., Suzaki, T., Kobayashi, S., Abe, K., and Ogata, E. (1984): <u>Biochem–Biophys. Res. Commun</u>. 119:212–219.
27. Klingenberg, M. (1961): <u>Biochem. Z</u>. 335:263–272.
28. Klingenberg, M. (1969): In: <u>The Energy Level and Metabolic Control in Mitochondria</u>, edited by S. Papa, J.M. Tager, E. Quagliariello, and E.C. Slater, pp. 189–193. Adriatic Editrice,   .
29. Koretsky, A.P., Wang, S., Murphy–Boesch, J., Klein, M.P., James, T.L., and Weiner, M.W. (1983): <u>Proc. Natl. Acad. Sci</u>. 80:7491–7495.
30. Lawson, J.W.R. and Veech, R.L. (1979): <u>J. Biol. Chem</u>. 254:6528–6537.
31. Leigh, Jr., J.S. and Chance, B. (1985): <u>Biophys. J</u>. 47:199.
32. Lemasters, J.J. (1984): <u>J. Biol. Chem</u>. 259:13123–13130.
33. Lynen, F. and Koenigsberger, R. (1951): <u>Ann. Chem</u>. 573:60–84.
34. Maruyama, K. and Weber, A. (1972): <u>Biochemistry</u> 11:2990–2998.
35. Nageswara Rao, B.D. and Cohn, M. (1981): <u>J. Biol. Chem</u>. 256:1716–1721.
36. Nioka, S., Chance, B., Subramanian, H., Hilberman, M., Richardson, M., and Egan, J. (1984): <u>"Metabolic Brain Death" in a Servo–Controlled Energy State of an Animal Model</u>. News of Metabolic Research, Vol 1, University of Pennsylvania, Phila, Pa., pp. 15–18.
37. Siesjo, B.K. (1978): <u>Brain Energy Metabolism</u>. John Wiley, New York.
38. Szent Gyorgyi, A.G. and Prior, G. (1966): <u>J. Mol. Biol</u>. 15:515–538.
39. Watson, W.E. (1976): <u>Cell Biology of Brain</u>. John Wiley and Sons,New York.
40. Weber, A., Heiz, R., and Reiss, I. (1969): <u>Biochemistry</u> 8:2266–2270.
41. Wu, R. and Racker, E. (1959): <u>J. Biol. Chem</u>. 234:1036–1041.

NMR in Biology and Medicine,
edited by Shu Chien and Chien Ho.
Raven Press, New York © 1986.

Cellular Biochemistry in Animals and Man Observed by ^{31}P NMR Spectroscopy*

George K. Radda and Shu Chien

Department of Biochemistry, University of Oxford, OX1 3QU, UK.

INTRODUCTION

The field of ^{31}P NMR spectroscopy began ten years ago and has since developed very quickly. It started with a relatively conventional spectrometer in 1974, with a probe size of only 8 mm (1). This system was used to obtain the phosphorus spectrum of skeletal muscle (Fig. 1). This gave us sufficient impetus to try to increase the size of the magnet and to take a much larger sample tubes, thus making it possible to perfuse an organ such as the heart and to maintain it within the probe. The spectrum

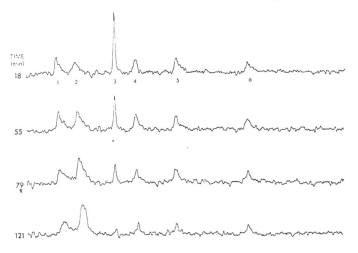

FIG. 1. ^{31}P Spectra of rat leg muscle at 129 MHz. Pulse interval 16 s, 50 scans. 1: sugar phosphate; 2: inorganic phosphate; 3: phosphocreatine; 4: γATP; 5: βATP; 6: αATP. From (1).

---

1 This paper is based on a lecture delivered by GKR and put in manuscript form by SC (Dept. of Physiology and Cellular Biophysics, Columbia Univ. College of Physicians and Surgeons, New York, NY 10032, U.S.A.

could then be obtained in about 1 min of accumulation time from a physiologically well maintained, beating rat heart. The subsequent development of the surface coil allowed the investigation of parts of a whole animal (2). In combination with methods to focus the observation in different parts of a live animal, so–called topical magnetic resonance, it became possible to study different organs within live animals by 1980–81 (3). The magnet that we now have for spectroscopy of human organs in whole body studies at Oxford is one with 1.9 Tesla. The history of the developement shows that from the frist obseration in 1974 we have progressed to human application remarkably rapidly in 8–9 years (Fig. 2).

In order to coordinate oxidative phosphorylation, phosphocreatine (PCr) utilization, and anaerobic glycogenolysis, there are mechanisms for switching from one to the other and for controlling the different pathways, as well as the delivery of oxygen and substrates through blood flow in the whole body. With NMR spectroscopy, we are able to study these pathways in humans as well as in animals. Although PCr has been described as an energy buffer, it has been suggested by Saks and others (4) that perhaps creatine kinase provides not only the buffer but also a shuttle between mitochondrially generated ATP and cytoplasmically required ATP in that there are two creatine kinase isoenzymes: one bound to the mitochondrial inner membrane and the other in the cytoplasm. The rapid conversion of ADP preferentially at the mitochondrial membrane might provide an extra mechanism for delivering energy from the mitochondria rapidly to the cytoplasm. Thus, the two main suggested roles of creatine kinase are as an energy buffer and as an energy shuttle. There is a third, and probably the most important, role for creatine kinase in controlling the level of ADP, which is important in determining the rates of both oxidative phosphorylation and glycolysis.

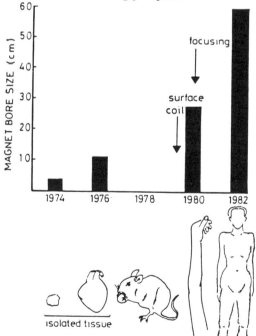

FIG. 2. Diagram showing the development of NMR spectroscopy from 1974 in terms of the magnet bore size (upper part) and the range of application from isolated tissues to whole body (lower part).

THE USE OF ³¹P SPECTROSCOPY TO STUDY MUSCLE METABOLISM

Our philosophy in performing the clinical studies is to devise very simple tests so that the duration of study can be minimized. Usually we need some kind of stress test with which the metabolic response to the stress and the subsequent recovery can be examined. We need to study what are the variations among normal individuals so that it is possible to determine what is abnormal in various disease states. In addition, in order to further our understanding of the clinical alterations, parallel animal models are needed to conduct the kinds of experiments that are not possible in human. Fig. 3 shows the type of study that has been performed

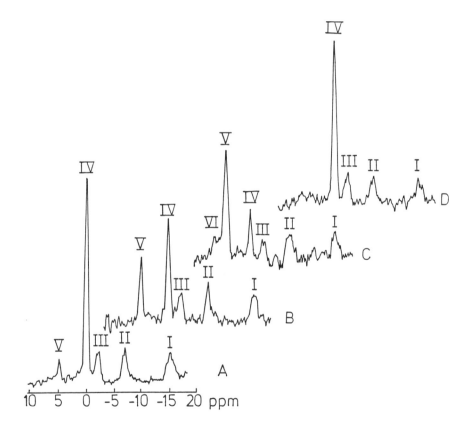

FIG. 3. Spectra from a subject before (A), during (B,C), and after (D) exercise. Exercise was carried out for 19 min to a pressure of 300mm Hg. Spectrum B was collected during the first min of exercise and C during the last min. D was obtained 5-6 min after exercise ceased. Spectrum A was collected over 256 s and all others over 64 s. Spectra are plotted as signal intensity against ppm, where ppm is the fractional frequency shift and the phosphocreatine signal is assigned a value of 0. Peak assignments are 1: β-ATP; II: α-ATP plus pyridine nucleotides; III: γ-ATP; IV: phospho-creatine; V: P_i; VI: phosphomonoesters. From (5).

in human using the small spectrometer, with a surface coil placed over the flexor digitorium superficialis muscle on the forearm. One can obtain the ³¹P NMR spectra at rest, during exercise, and during recovery.

One of the problems is that the individual variations of normals in their response to exercise is large. For example, there are differences in the relation of work to the ratio of phosphocratine to inorganic phosphate (PCr/P_i) as a result of training. More importantly, one can see large variations in the amount of glycogen used compared to the oxidative rate at the initial phase of exercise in terms of pH changes, the amount of PCr used, etc. In order to use ³¹P–NMR spectroscopy as a clinical tool to detect abnormalities, then we clearly need to be able to define parameters that are reasonably invariant from individual to individual. There are three constant parameters that will be used in the ensuing discussions in relation to disease states (5). The first of these is the relationship between PCr utilization and change in intracellular pH (pH_i), i.e. the acidification by lactate production (Fig. 4). We find in several hundred control subjects that the shape of this curve is extremely constant, showing that glycogenolysis is turned on very rapidly only after about 60–70% of the PCr has already been used. Thus, this constant relationship represents the control point for turning on glycogenolysis in relation to demand, which is perhaps indicated by how much PCr has been used. The second parameter is the rapid rate of PCr resynthesis, which has a half–time of about 1 min (there is a slower component related to pH changes) following the period of aerobic or anaerobic exercise (Fig. 5). This parameter represents the controlled rate of oxidative phosphorylation in the recovering muscle. The

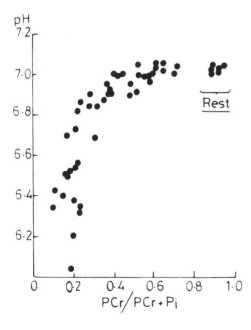

FIG. 4. Relationship between the ratio $PCr/(PCr+P_i)$ and intracellular pH in normal control subjects undergoing exercise. The 6 points on the right were obtained at rest. Modified from (5).

third invariant parameter is the rate of recovery of pH$_i$ to its original level after exercise (Fig. 6), reaching a level which is variable among individuals. This recovery rate, which has a half–time of about 6 min, represents the rate at which lactate is washed out from the muscle. Using these parameters, we can detect abnormalities that fall outside the normal ranges.

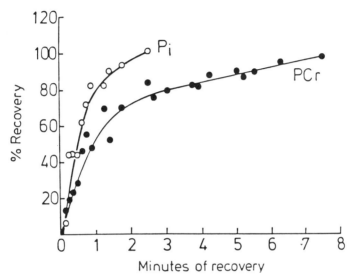

FIG. 5. Rates of recovery of P$_i$ and PCr following exercise. Data from (5).

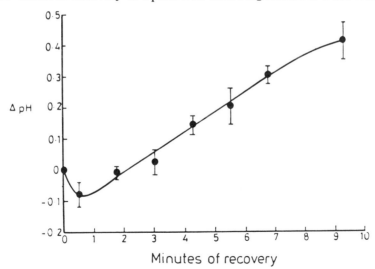

FIG. 6. The rate of recovery of pH$_i$ following exercise. The data of pH$_i$ change (ΔpH) are plotted with reference to the lowest level reached at the end of the exercise period. Data from (5).

In our protocol, the arm of the subject is placed in the magnet, and the magnetic field homogeneity is adjusted by shimming on the protons of the water and fat in the arm. This takes 1–2 min. Thereafter an initial ^{31}P spectrum is collected in 1 min, and then a spectrum is collected for 4 min, with 128 scans, so that pH_i can be measured accurately. The subject is then asked to perform some light, aerobic, dynamic exercise by squeezing a rubber bulb, initially at a pressure of 100 mmHg, for about 4 min; most patients, however weak, can do that exercise. In order to stress the stronger people, the pressure is increased to 300 mmHg and the patient is asked to continue the exercise up to about 3 min. Following these two periods of exercises, the recovery phase is studied for about 15 min. During the whole period of examination of about 35 min, some 30 spectra are collected which can be analyzed for concentrations, pH and other relationships to be described below.

STUDIES ON MUSCLE DISEASES

Over the first 2 1/2 years we have studied over 300 patients and carried out more than 600 examinations of a variety of muscle diseases and other diseases which are reflected in the metabolism of the muscle (Table I). These results show that we now have a tool for the non–invasive study of biochemistry in vivo. This table, which was prepared in March 1984, serves

Table I. Patient Census (1 March 1984, total 270)

Metabolic Myopathies (Phosphorylase, Debrancher, PFK,
Phosphorylase kinase, Acid Maltase)   15

Mitochondrial Myopathies   15

Dystrophy (Duchenne, Dystrophia myotonica, Limb girdle,
Becker, Others, Carriers, Relatives)   38

Neuropathies (Brachial plexus lesion, Motor neurone disease
Spinal muscular atrophy, Others)   12

Systemic Disorders (Abnormal thyroid function,
Diabetes, Renal failure, Malnutrition)   38

Myositis, Myasthenia Gravis   3

Altered Plasma Ions (Pi ↑↓, Mg^{++} ↓, K^+ ↑↓)   24

Undiagnosed Muscle Problems PVS ± treatment (e.g. verapamil,
(menadione, ubiquinone, thyroxine)   70

Deficient O_2 Delivery (Anaemia ± transfusion, Thalassaemia, Sclero–
derma, Arterial oclusion, peripheral vascular disease)   30

Elderly Controls   12

to give a general indication that we have seen a whole range of patients with deficiencies in different enzymes, abnormal mitochrondria, and various forms of muscular dystrophy. For comparison, we have also carried out studies on a variety of neurophathies, some of whom (e.g. with brachial plexus lesions) can be studied before and after a reparative operation. Since muscle metabolism might be expected to reflect some of the systemic disorders, e.g. renal failure, these patients has been studied before and after treatment to see whether the metabolic changes in the muscle can be used as an index of the degree of correction of the abnormalities by procedures, e.g. renal dialysis. We studied a group of patients with abnormal plasma iron concentrations before and after treatment. We have addressed the questions whether a low phosphate in the blood is reflected in the phosphate handling by the muscle, and how a low magnesium in the blood affects muscle metabolism. We have also studied patients with undiagnosed muscle disorders who were referred to us because the clinicians were at a loss after having had an extensive series of tests. In many cases we have successful observations about various metabolic abnormalities, and we have been able to treat some of these patients with drugs and observe changes after the treatment. We will show some studies on patients with deficient oxygen delivery, particularly these with peripheral vascular disease. We have examined the relationship between oxidative metabolism and oxygen delivery in patients with thalassemia and other forms of abnormal hemoglobin oxygen carrying capacity.

In terms of muscle metabolism, we can study the diseases listed in Table I that affect various parts of the sequence of events shown in Fig. 7. Mitochondrial abnormalities can either inhibit the oxidative chain or

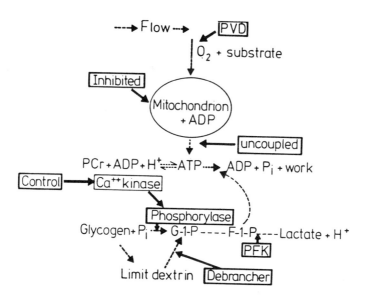

FIG. 7. Schematic diagram showing the bioenergetics of muscle and the points where abnormalities affect the metabolism.

uncouple the oxidation of substrate from ATP synthesis; we have seen patients in both groups. There is a whole group of patients in whom we believe the control functions of turning on glycogenolysis compared to the oxidative reaction is abnormal. As mentioned above, there are patients with deficiency of enzymes in the glycolytic sequence or related enzymes. With the use of a few examples, we will show how the non–invasive studies of these patients, who are effectively human mutants, can lead not only to an understanding of the actual condition of the individual, but also to the learning of new biochemistry.

First, we will show the results on patients with McArdle's syndrome, a disease with the absence of phosphorylase in muscle. Fig. 8 shows the results from one of the first patients we have studied. These patients get cramp during aerobic exercise. In constrast to normal individuals, who would start to produce lactic acid as soon as they use up 70% of their PCr (Fig. 4), these patients can not produce lactic acid, so their pH_i does not decrease but rather increases to ~7.3 as P_i builds up; at that point the patient can not continue to work and the muscle is severely cramped. If they keep on trying to exercise, they will go through the pain barrier and reach a "second wind", when they are able to exercise again. They can then increase the work load and gradually drop the intracellular pH back to normal, decreasing slightly the P_i and increasing their PCr. The time taken to reach the second wind is variable among patients. After the second wind they are able to go on working for a long period. This is a systemic effect related to the increased substrate delivery to the muscle, because if the patient reachs the second wind with his right arm, his left arm does not go through the cramp phase, the alkalinization, etc., but is able to work in the same way as if it had already gone through the same protocol.

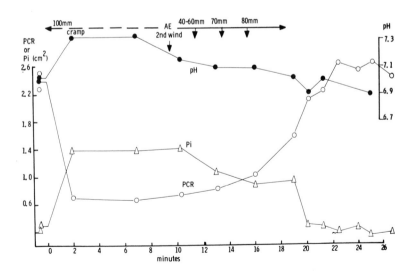

FIG. 8.   Showing the effects of aerobic exercise on pH_i, P_i and PCr in a patient with McArdle's syndrome.

By studying these patients, we have been able to investigate the role of ADP in controlling muscle function, and this turns out to be very important. If one uses the creatine kinase reaction to calculate, from the equilibrium constant, the concentration of ADP and takes note of the fact that [H⁺] is part of the equation, then it can be shown that normal individuals, during light or heavy exercise, only increase their ADP from the resting level of ~10 µM to somewhere in the range of 40–80 µM. In contrast, patients with McArdle's syndrome increase their intracellular ADP to 240 or even 300 µM during the cramp period, but drop down to 80–100 µM when they have reached the second wind. These patients cannot increase their H⁺ concentration, which serves to counterbalance the increase in ADP concentration during exercise, and they build up an usually high ADP level (Fig. 9). In muscle, ADP increases the rate of oxidative phosphorylation, so it is a positive effector of oxidation; at the same time it is a negative effector of contractility because it inhibits the myosin ATPase. Therefore, it is important to keep the ADP level in a delicate balance between that being able to stimulate oxidation in relation to the demand and that not inhibiting the ATPase too much if work is to be continued.

The rate of oxidative phosphorylation in the muscle can be measured from the rate of PCr resynthesis following the period of exercise. In comparison to normal individuals, patients with McArdle's syndrome increase their ADP to higher levels and have a more rapid PCr resynthesis. A Langmuir–Burke plot of the initial rate of PCr resynthesis (1/v) against the calculated ADP concentration can be used to determine the K_m and V_{max} for mitochondrial oxidative phosphorylation in human muscle (Fig. 10). The K_m for ADP activation of oxidative phosphorylation in vivo is found to be 27 µM, which is a very reasonable number in comparison to the value in isolated mitochondria. Thus, by studying patients with abnormal conditions, we can learn about the control of various reactions in vivo.

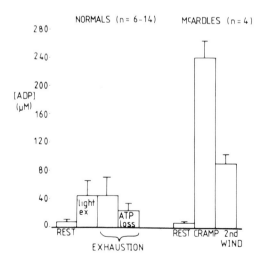

FIG. 9. ADP concentrations in exercising muscle of patients with McArdle's syndrome compared to normal controls, calculated from the creatine kinase equilibrium.

Fig. 11 illustrates a simplified version of the mitochondrial electron transport chain which is coupled through the H⁺ gradient to the synthesis of ATP. We have studied patients who have electron transport deficiencies either by not being able to use some of the substrates, or having a block pf a later stage e.g. at the cytochrome b level. We have also seen patients, who although are able to oxidize substrates rapidly, cannot use that

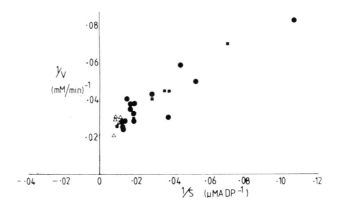

FIG. 10.   Langmuir–Burke plot of PCr recovery rates after exercise used to determine the K_m (27 μM) and V_{max} (43 mM min⁻¹) for mitochondrial oxidative phosphorylation in human muscle; ● control subjects after light exercise; ■ control subjects after heavy excersie; Δ patients with McArdle's disease.

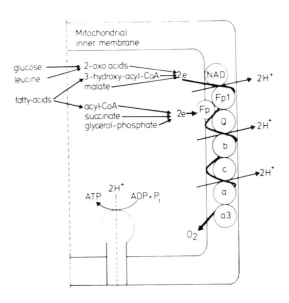

FIG. 11.   A simplified version of mitochondrial electron transport chain.

energy to convert efficiently to ATP. Among the first group we have reported the case of two sisters who both suffered from a block at the NADH coenzyme Q part of the electron transport chain; their rate of recovery from exercise in terms of PCr resynthesis is extremely slow (by a factor of 10) in comparison to control subjects (6).

Table II summarizes the 12 mitochondrial disorders we have studied. NMR detected some abnormalities in 11 of these patients. By measuring the [ATP]/[ADP][P$_i$] ratio in the resting muscle, we have found a low phosphorylation potential (usually by an order of magnitude lower than that in normal subjects) in 10 of the 12 patients who had known mitochondrial disorders on the basis of histology. The rate of PCr resynthesis was found to be slow in only 4 of the 12 mitochondrial disorders. This is because that, while mitochondrial function is severely stressed during exercise, it is not stressed to its maximum capacity during the recovery phase. This is shown by the fact that the rate of ADP recovery after exercise was slower than normal in 6 of the 12 patients. At the early stages of recovery (when ADP is rapidly rephosphorylated) mitochondrial activity is close to maximal.

We will present next some patients who show abnormalities in the control of glycogenolysis. Fig. 12 illustrates a case of a 30–year old man, who had a severe virus attack of chicken pox. In response to

Table II. Intracellular pH, phosporylation Potential, and recovery rates of pH$_i$, PCr and ADP in patients with mitochondrial myopathies

<u>Mitochondrial Myopathies</u>

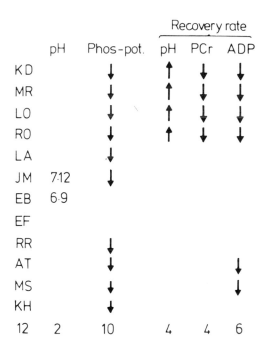

	pH	Phos-pot.	Recovery rate		
			pH	PCr	ADP
KD		↓	↑	↓	↓
MR		↓	↑	↓	↓
LO		↓	↑	↓	↓
RO		↓	↑	↓	↓
LA		↓			
JM	7.12	↓			
EB	6.9				
EF					
RR		↓			
AT		↓			↓
MS		↓			↓
KH		↓			
12	2	10	4	4	6

exercise, in contrast to normal control subjects who turns on glycogenolysis only after 60–70% of the PCr has been used, this patient turns on glycogenolysis almost immediately and acidifies extremely rapidly. We have seen this condition in 14 patients, whose pH change in response to exercise indicates a much more rapid acidification than control subjects. These patients all had post–viral muscle fatigue (7). Therefore, we are now able to study new kinds of diseases that, perhaps, were not accessible to medical investigations until the availability of a non–invasive tool that can be used to examine the dynamics of events and the control of metabolism within the living system.

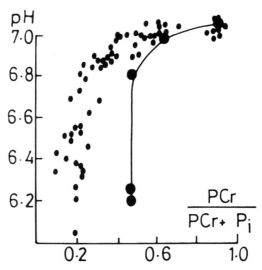

FIG. 12. The relationship between pH_i and the ratio $PCr/(PCr+P_i)$ in the muscle during exercise of a patient with post–viral exhaustion/fatigue syndrome (large dots, solid line); control subjects: small dots. Modified from (7).

STUDIES ON PERIPHERAL VASCULAR DISEASES

Our whole body system at the John Radcliffe Hospital, which has been operational for less than a year, has a magnet operating at 1.9 Tesla; this special clinical facility allows us to look at spectroscopy of any part of human body with varying degrees of success. First we will present the results of studies on peripheral vascular disease. The patient is placed in the magnet with a surface coil positioned under the calf muscle; then he is asked to exercise within the magnet by peddling against the prescribed weight. The weight that the patient worked against was determined on the basis of his lean body mass. We followed changes both during work, which lasted for about 10 min, and the recovery phase. We can see similar spectral changes during work as in the arm: using up PCr, retaining the ATP level, and acidifying as seen from the shift of P_i, and we can follow the rate of recovery. Fourteen patients with claudication, i.e. exercise–induced pain in the lower limb, were compared to control subjects during a 10–min period of exercise. The claudicants can be divided into two groups on the basis of their symptoms and clinical studies, e.g. ankle Doppler measurements, into severe and less severe groups. The PCr utilization for all severe claudicants, who were unable to complete the 10 min period of exercise because of pain, was larger than that for the control mean by more than 2 S.D. The results on less severe claudicants generally fell below the control mean, but not by more than 2 S.D. Similarly, the pH decreased more in the severe claudicants than in control subjects during exercise. The severe claudicants also had a slower recovery in pH, showing that the severe limitation in blood flow causes lactate washout to be very slow. In a severe claudicant who preoperatively was only able to complete 3 min of exercise, the pH_i decreased to 6.6 (control 7.0). Postoperatively, the patient was able to exercise to 10 min, and the pH_i change was much smaller, being within the normal range. What is interesting in this study is that, although the blood flow recovered immediately after the operation,the recovery in metabolic function took a week or two. Apparently there are adoptive changes associated with the impaired oxygen delivery that took same time to reverse.

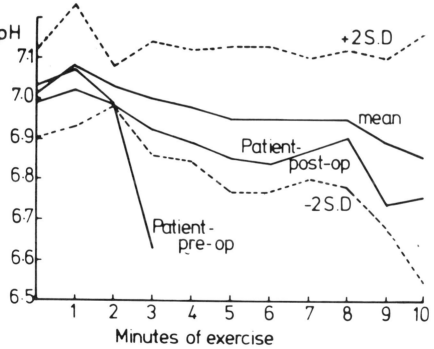

FIG. 13. pH changes in gastrocnemius muscle during exercise in control subjects and in a patient with intermittent claudication. Mean represents control subjects and the dotted lines show 2 standard deviations of these. Patient pre–op refers to changes seen before operation and post–op after femoral artery by–pass. Study done by Hands, Galloway, Bore, Morris and Radda.

STUDIES ON THE BRAIN

Our studies on the brain were performed with the use of a 600 mm bore magnet which initially operated at 1.6T. We place a surface coil on the head of the patient, and we are able to look at the brain using the field profiling method to eliminate contributions from the muscle. In field profiling, we shape the static magnetic field in such a way that it is only homogeneous within a given volume element which can be closed down to an approximate sphere of about 4 cm in diameter. By locating that sphere inside the head, we can collect the signal from the human brain. The upper part of Fig. 14 shows a spectrum from a normal control subject. This spectrum was manipulated to remove the very broad component collected from the signal in the bone phosphates. Because of the manipulation of the spectrum one distorts the observed ratios and sometimes even the positions of the signals, and one must be very careful in deriving precise quantitative conclusions from such manipulated spectra. But there are various tricks, one of which will be discussed later, that can be used to circumvent this problem. The PCr to ATP ratio in this subject is about 1.5 to 1, with allowance made for the effects of relaxations. In addition to ATP and PCr, there is a large component in adult human brain from the phosphodiester region, and unlike in the neonatal human brain shown by Dr. Dawson at this Symposium, we do not see a large peak in the phosphomonoester region. The phosphodiester peak is of interest in relation to some demyelination diseases which we have began to study, but for most purposes it is a nuisance because it hides the P_i that one would like to use to derive the pH_i. The lower part of Fig. 14 shows the spectrum of a patient with a

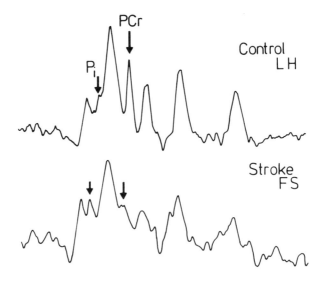

FIG. 14. ³¹P NMR Spectra of human brain at 1.6T obtained by using the field profiling method. Upper spectrum was obtained from a normal control subject; lower spectrum from a patient with a stroke on his right side. (Study carried out by Galloway, Hilton–Jones, Rajagopalan, Radda).

fairly superficial, large stroke on his right side. There is a dramatic decrease in the PCr peak, an overall decrease of the signal–to–noise ratio, and an increase in P_i.

We have studied three patients with strokes and they differ in some respects. The interesting observations are in the two patients labelled JR and FS (Fig. 15). In JR the stroke resulted in a large decrease in the PCr/P_i ratio, but no change in the PCr/ATP, and hence also a decrease in ATP/P_i. FS is different in that PCr/P_i ratio decreased, and so did PCr/ATP. Thus, in JR the brain regions studied consist of either entirely dead cells (containing P_i and virtually no PCr and ATP) or entirely normal cells, whereas in FS the ratio of PCr/P_i may reflect a mixture of normal and dead cells. These differences may be related to the duration of the stroke, but these are only two studies in this early stage of our investigations.

The patient labelled CH is not a stroke patient, but this case is unusual in that it was solved on the basis of ³¹P–NMR and not the standard clinical tools. A girl (age 15) has been known since the age of 9 to have some kind of cerebral disorders, based on the history of convulsion and other manifestations. CT scan of her brain showed generalized atrophy and dense spots at the basal ganglia that were ascribed to calcification. Four years of clinical studies pointed to some undiagnosed brain disorder, possibly vasculitis. During a clinical presentation, the neurologist who has been associated with our NMR program observed that she could not stand very easily from her chair and recommended detailed muscle studies to see if there was also muscle involvement. The initial resting muscle spectrum showed that the phosphorylation potential was 10 fold lower than normal controls; hence we suspected some form of mitochondrial myopathy. This was confirmed by muscle biopsy which showed mitochondria with abnormal

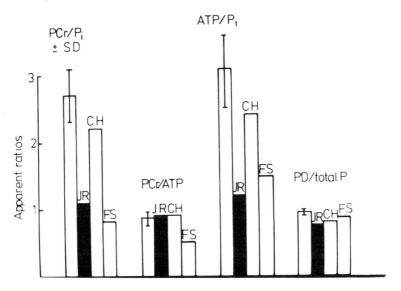

FIG. 15. Apparent ratios of PCr/P_i, PCr/ATP, ATP/P_i and PD/total P in three patients (JR, CH and FS) compared with normal controls (left most bar in each group showing mean ± S.D.).

appearance, and studies on the individual reactions of the mitochondria isolated from the biopsy demonstrated a block at the NADH coenzyme Q reductase. Her brain spectrum showed an elevated level of P_i and a decrease of PCr; these changes mirrored those in the resting muscle. Therefore, we concluded that she had the same mitochondrial disorder in her brain as in her muscle.

STUDIES ON THE LIVER

One of the problems in studying internal organs such as the human liver is how well can the observation be focused. If a surface coil is placed over the abdomen of the patient, one detects the signal from PCr as well as ATP, although the liver does not contain PCr. The method of focusing involves the adjustment of the homogeneous volume to a region where one no long detects any PCr signal. If one uses a 10 cm surface probe and initially looks at a volume of about 10 cm in diameter, the abdominal muscle will be included in the signal. By reducing the volume progressively to 4 cm in diameter, one can bring the detection range to the inside of the body and obtain the pure liver spectrum of a fasting, healthy human volunteer. The ratio of sugar phosphate to ATP and P_i/ATP can be quantitated from the ratio of peak areas, because the relaxation times are very short in the liver (Table III). The pH_i in the human liver is about 7.18.

Liver function tests can be designed in which the metabolic function of the liver is stressed. When fructose is infused into an individual, it is converted to fructose–1–phosphate by fructose kinase, and the enzyme aldolase B breaks it down to glyceraldehyde and dihydroxyacetone–P; from there it goes on to generate glucose and lactate (Fig. 16). This is an ATP utilizing reaction. There are conditions where patients are intolerant to fructose or other sugars, e.g. galactose. If a healthy volunteer receives 200 mg/kg of fructose infusion, by studying the liver spectrum before and at various time intervals after the infusion (e.g., 5, 10, 15 min, etc.), one can follow the time course of the buildup of the fructose–1–phosphate, its reutilization, and the changes of the P_i level (Fig. 17). The time course

Table III.   Reproducibility of ³¹P Magnetic Resonance Spectroscopy of Liver in Seven Healthy Subjects*

Mean ± SEM

$$\frac{\text{Sugar–P}}{\beta\text{ATP}} = 0.53 \pm 0.03$$

Ratio of peak areas

$$\frac{P_i}{\beta\text{ATP}} = 0.97 \pm 0.04$$

$$pH = 7.18 \pm 0.03$$

*Results obtained by Oberhansli, Galloway, Taylor, Bore and Radda.

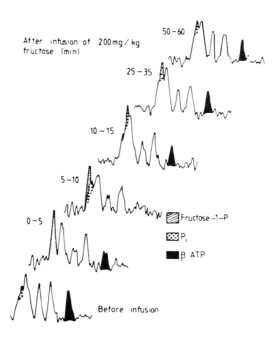

After infusion of 200mg/kg fructose (min)

50 - 60

25 - 35

10 - 15

5 - 10

0 - 5

Fructose -1-P

P$_i$

β ATP

Before infusion

FIG. 17. The liver spectra of a healthy volunteer obtained before and at various time intervals (numbers in minutes indicated next to the spectra) after receiving 200 mg/kg of fructose infusion, showing the time course of changes of fructose-1-phosphate, P$_i$ level and βATP. (Experiments by Oberhansli, Galloway, Taylor, Bore and Radda, to be published).

the abdomen, with spectra generated at 8 mm slices as one progresses inward from the skin towards the liver. The skin has no phosphate, next the muscle spectrum is detected, then the muscle signal decreases and one progresses more and more to the spectrum of the liver. This study took 45 min, but now we can speed up the observation. This method will allow better spectroscopic localization in human subjects.

FUTURE PERSPECTIVES

Next, we would like to discuss what the future might hold in the way of promise. By using a special surface coil we can obtain a spectrum from an adult human heart showing a large signal for the 2,3-diphosphoglycerate in the blood going through the left ventricle; this would not be seen in the skeletal muscle. The PCr/ATP ratio is about 2, and that took 4 min to accummulate. One is thus able to begin to consider looking at various conditions of the heart. There are other forms of measurements that can be made in addition to the steady state concentrations. For example, the

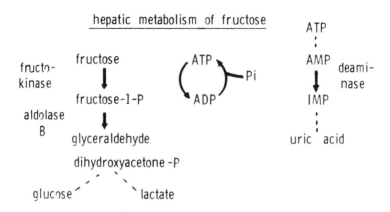

FIG. 16. Schematic diagram summarizing the pathways for hepatic metabolism of fructose.

shows an initial buildup of the sugar phosphates, and this is followed by a fairly rapid decrease back to control. The fructose concentration in the plasma measured simultaneously also reflects these changes. The significant decrease in [ATP] and its slow recovery shows that the liver is not able to control its ATP level nearly as well as muscle and other organs. The most surprising finding is the handling of the inorganic phosphate. The initial rapid drop in P_i, which is expected, shows that the transfer of P_i from the plasma volume into the liver is too slow to replenish that is needed for the phosphorylation reaction. But after the sugar phosphate has been hydrolyzed back and the phosphate has been regenerated, the high level of the P_i compared to the control is maintained for over 1 hr. Thus, the liver cannot clear the high P_i level during that period; it has a lower ATP, high P_i, and presumably very low phosphorylation potential for a long time after such a stress test. Quite clearly this test enables one to study diseases of the liver that are associated with metabolic disorders involving one of these functions.

In order to focus the spectroscopic observation, ideally one would like to have some form of imaging trick and use it to achieve better localization. One method is the so-called rotating frame imaging, where one uses the properties of B1 field gradient to spatially label the location of the signal (8). One can achieve a B1 field gradient by using the surface coil as the B1 field decreases with distance away from the coil. To perform such studies, one uses a large transmitter coil which is concentric with a slightly displaced smaller receiver coil; the two coils are electrically decoupled so that they do not communicate with each other (9). In this manner, one has a linear B1 field gradient and a sensitive volume from which signal can be picked up which is defined by this small surface coil (Fig. 18). Imaging experiments can thus be performed to yield slices of about 8 mm in thickness and 4 cm in diameter, which is the size of the inner surface coil, going in toward the patient (10). Fig. 19 shows a study on the human liver with such a double surface coil placed over

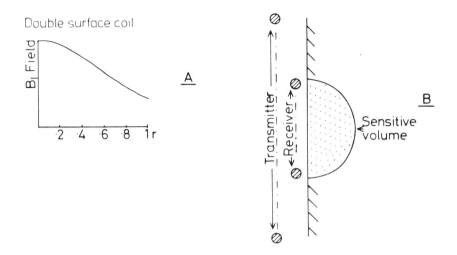

FIG. 18. A: The field strength along the axis of a surface coil. B: A cross section through the double surface–coil probe showing the relative position of transmitter and receiver coil and the sensitive volume within the sample. From (10).

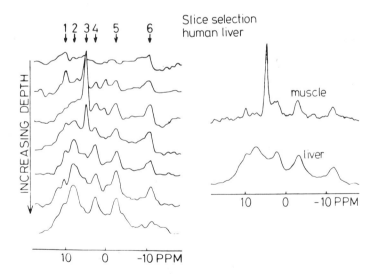

FIG. 19. (A) The set of spatially localized ^{31}P spectra from the thorax of a human subject obtained by rotating frame imaging. Peak assignments: (1) inorganic phosphate; (2) phosphodiesters; (3) phosphocreatine; (4,5,6) adenosine triphosphate. (B) A spectrum of human skeletal muscle obtained with a surface coil. (C) A spectrum of human liver obtained with a surface coil in conjunction with the method of field profiling. (Spectrum C by courtesy of Drs. G. Galloway, R. Oberhansli, and D. Taylor). From (10).

saturation transfer method can be used to measure reaction fluxes both at equilibrium and steady state. In this method, one of the peaks, e.g. the γ phosphate of the ATP, is saturated and then one observes the extent to which this saturation is chemically transferred either to PCr or P_i manifested as a decrease in the signal intensity of the appropriate peaks related to the unidirectional fluxes of PCr → ATP or P_i → ATP and to the relaxation time of these peaks (Fig. 20). For a beating, isolated rat heart, the PCr → ATP flux is about 5 times that of the ATP synthesis rate, showing that creatine kinase is more rapid and is in equilibrium. However, this system of energy backup is not necessary for the proper functioning of the heart, as shown by animal experiments in which the metabolism was altered. Over 90% of the PCr in a rat was replaced by an analogue, β–guanidino–propionic acid (β-GPA), which led to the generation of phosphoguanidino–propionic acid (PGPA), which is a poor substrate for creatine kinase. PGPA reacts 1000 times more slowly than PCr, and hence cannot provide the rapid backup energy as PCr. ^{31}P-NMR studies on the isolated, perfused heart of rats fed β-GPA for two weeks showed a marked decrease in PCr peak. The rate of PCr → ATP conversion can be studied with the saturation transfer method. In normal controls, the flux of PCr was 10 sec^{-1} as compared to the rate of ATP synthesis and utilization of about 3 sec   (Table IV). With β-GPA, the flux of PCr was reduced to 2 sec^{-1}, which is below the rate of ATP utilization, and yet the heart functioned normally, reacted appropriately to stress and maintained the ATP levels within the same narrow range as normal, despite the presence of a very small amount of PCr (11). Therefore the presence of the control function, even in the absence of energy backup function, allows the heart to function normally. We are currently investigating the intricate details of this metabolic control.

Another direction of future developments is other forms of spectroscopy. Fig. 21 shows the naturally abundant ^{13}C NMR spectrum

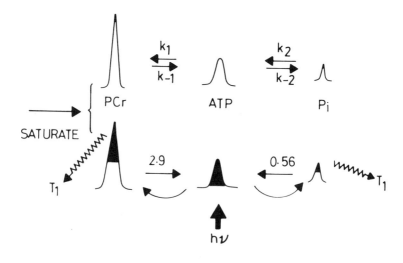

FIG. 20. Use of the saturation transfer to measure reaction fluxes.

saturation transfer method can be used to measure reaction fluxes both at equilibrium and steady state. In this method, one of the peaks, e.g. the γ phosphate of the ATP, is saturated and then one observes the extent to which this saturation is chemically transferred either to PCr or P_i manifested as a decrease in the signal intensity of the appropriate peaks related to the unidirectional fluxes of PCr → ATP or P_i → ATP and to the relaxation time of these peaks (Fig. 20). For a beating, isolated rat heart, the PCr → ATP flux is about 5 times that of the ATP synthesis rate, showing that creatine kinase is more rapid and is in equilibrium. However, this system of energy backup is not necessary for the proper functioning of the heart, as shown by animal experiments in which the metabolism was altered. Over 90% of the PCr in a rat was replaced by an analogue, β–guanidino–propionic acid (β–GPA), which led to the generation of phosphoguanidino–propionic acid (PGPA), which is a poor substrate for creatine kinase. PGPA reacts 1000 times more slowly than PCr, and hence cannot provide the rapid backup energy as PCr. ^{31}P–NMR studies on the isolated, perfused heart of rats fed β–GPA for two weeks showed a marked decrease in PCr peak. The rate of PCr → ATP conversion can be studied with the saturation transfer method. In normal controls, the flux of PCr was 10 sec^{-1} as compared to the rate of ATP synthesis and utilization of about 3 sec^{-1} (Table IV). With β–GPA, the flux of PCr was reduced to 2 sec^{-1}, which is below the rate of ATP utilization, and yet the heart functioned normally, reacted appropriately to stress and maintained the ATP levels within the same narrow range as normal, despite the presence of a very small amount of PCr (11). Therefore the presence of the control function, even in the absence of energy backup function, allows the heart to function normally. We are currently investigating the intricate details of this metabolic control.

Another direction of future developments is other forms of spectroscopy. Fig. 21 shows the naturally abundant ^{13}C NMR spectrum

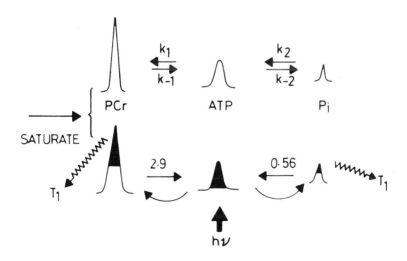

FIG. 20. Use of the saturation transfer to measure reaction fluxes.

Table IV. CPK Saturation Transfer in Working Hearts*

$\frac{M+}{M^0}$	Tim (s)	T₁ (s)	K (s^{-1})	[PCr] ($\frac{mmol}{g\ dry}$)	Flux ([ ]s^{-1})	RPP ($\frac{mmHg}{min}$ $\times 10^{-3}$)	$-\dot{V}O_2$ ([ ]s^{-1})	ATPase ([ ]s^{-1})
Controls 0.36 ±0.05	1.5 ±0.1	4.3 ±1.0	0.45 ±0.01	22.2	10.0	27.3 ±1.8	0.5	3.4
GPA–Fed 0.22 ±0.08		4.5	0.81	2.5	2.0	22.5 ±1.3	0.4	2.7
Sum (0.19)			(0.95)		(2.4)			

(T₁ PGPA = 5.3±0.1 s)

* From (1).

taken from a part of the fat on the abdomen in a very lean individual in the whole human spectrometer. By using a selective form of decoupling, one can quantitatively measure the ratio of saturated to polyunsaturated fats in about 10 min. This non–invasive method would be valuable since the extent of fat composition has been related to various forms of diseases, not the least coronary heart disease and patients at risk for this disease.

The last point we will discuss is to return to the method of cleaning up the spectrum. In the future we may be able to use all the tricks organic chemists have used, to study spectra within the human body. In the brain spectrum shown in Fig. 22, such cleaning up allows us to pick up the relevant components such as PCr and P$_i$ from overlapping peaks such as the phosphodiester. When one does the spin–echo experiment, the spectrum is already cleaned up to some extent. If in addition to spin–echo, one performs a selective J–coupling experiment by radiating the proton next to the phosphate groups in a special may, the signals from those components that have protons coupled to the phosphorus are abolished. In such an experiment, one can completely eliminate the signal from the phosphodiester region, and thus the PCr/P$_i$ ratio can be determined without any interference, and the pH$_i$ can be determined much more accurately from a single peak than as a shoulder on a large component (12).

In summary, there are both medical information and new tricks in spectroscopy that will take us a long way to investigate human metabolism in disease states and in normal subjects.

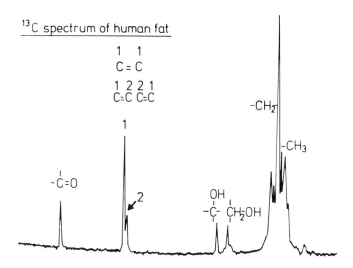

FIG. 21. ¹³C NMR spectrum taken from a part of the fat on the abdomen in whole human spectrometer (Oberhansli and Galloway, unpublished).

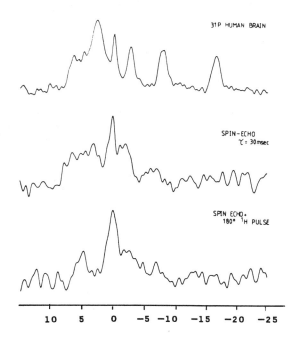

FIG. 22. Spin–echo and J–modulated ³¹P spectra of human brain. For details see (12).

ACKNOWLEDGMENTS

The work described has had many contributors, and in this form they cannot be given the credit they deserve. Since the lecture, however, several of the studies have been published and these publications give the appropriate credits. Financial support for the work has been largely from the Medical Research Council, the British Heart Foundation, the Department of Heath and Social Security and the National Institutes of Health.

REFERENCES

1. Hoult, D.I., Busby, S.J.W., Gadian, D.G., Radda, G.K., Richards, R.E. and Seeley, P.J. (1974): Nature 252:285–287.
2. Ackerman, J.J.H., Grove, T.H., Wong, G.G., Gadian, D.G. and Radda, G.K. (1980): Nature 283:167–170.
3. Gordon, R.E., Hanley, P.E., Shaw, D., Gadian, D.G., Radda, G.K., Styles, P., Bore, P.J. and Chan, L. (1980): Nature 287:367–368.
4. Saks, V.A., Rosenshtrautch, L.V., Smirnov, V.N. and Chazov, E.I. (1978): Canad. J. Physiol. Pharmacol. 56:691–706.
5. Taylor, D.J., Bore, P.J., Styles, P., Gadian, D.G. and Radda, G.K. (1983): Mol. Biol. Med. 1:77–94.
6. Radda, G.K., Bore, P.J., Gadian, D.G., Ross, B.D., Styles, P, Taylor, D.J. and Morgan–Hughes, J. (1982): Nature 295:608–609.
7. Arnold, D.L., Bore, P.J., Radda, G.K., Styles, P. and Taylor, D.J. (1984): Lancet i:1367–1369.
8. Hoult, D.I. (1979): J. Magn. Reson. 33:183–197.
9. Styles, P., Smith, M.B., Briggs, R.W. and Radda, G.K. (1985): J. Magn. Reson. 62, 397–405.
10. Styles, P., Scott, C.A. and Radda, G.K. (1985): J. Magn. Reson. 2:402–409.
11. Shoubridge, E.A., Jeffry, F.M.H., Keogh, J.M., Radda, G.K. and Seymour, A.-M. L. (1985): Biochim. Biophys. Acta 847:25–32
12. Brindle, K.M., Smith M.B., Rajagopalan, B. and Radda, G. K. (1985): J. Magn. Reson. 61:559–563.

NMR in Biology and Medicine,
edited by Shu Chien and Chien Ho.
Raven Press, New York © 1986.

Concluding Remarks

Shu Chien

*Department of Physiology and Cellular Biophysics, Columbia University College
of Physicians and Surgeons, New York, New York 10032*

The primary goals of this symposium are to introduce new concepts and technology in NMR to the Republic of China in Taiwan and to promote the interactions between investigators here and abroad, with the ultimate aim of applying this new technology to advance biomedical research and to improve health care. This symposium has succeeded in meeting these goals.

A major mission of the sponsoring institutions, i.e. the Central Laboratory of Molecular Biology and the Institute of Biomedical Sciences of Academia Sinica and the National Science Council, is to promote research studies on the structure and function of living organisms at various levels, including molecules, cells, organs and systems, both in health and in disease. This symposium shows that NMR provides us with the unique capabilities to gain new insights into the structure and function of living organisms at all these levels.

The Symposium consisted of four sessions. Drs. Chien Ho, Myer Bloom and Robert Griffin spoke at the first session on Solid–State NMR Studies of Biological Systems. Drs. Aksel Bothner–By, Sunney Chan, Paul Ts'o and Brian Reid were the speakers at the second session on High–Resolution NMR of Biological Macromolecules. With a combination of elegant experimental studies and sophisticated theoretical analysis, these speakers of the first two sessions have shown us how NMR can be used to elucidate the molecular structure and dynamic interactions of lipids, proteins and nucleic acids in solutions, solid state and cellular systems. These studies have provided fundamental knowledge in molecular biology and cell biology that has not been attainable by other approaches.

The papers of the third session on NMR imaging were given by Drs. Paul Lauterbur, Harry Genant and Ralph Alfidi. Their lucid lectures on the principles and application of NMR imaging and their beautiful illustrations of the NMR images in a variety of conditions have demonstrated to us how the detailed structures of organ systems in the body can be visualized by this new technique under normal and pathological states. They also informed us of the exciting new developments and great future potentials in NMR imaging.

In the fourth session on in vivo NMR spectroscopy, Drs. Joan Dawson, John Leigh and George Radda showed us the ingenious approaches they have developed in which NMR spectroscopy is used to study non–invasively energy metabolism and cellular biochemistry in various organs and tissues of animals and man. Their lectures clearly illustrate that in vivo NMR spectroscopy is a powerful technique for elucidating metabolic functions in normal conditions and their derangement in pathological states.

In summary, the presentations in these four sessions on the use of NMR to study biological systems from molecules to man have shed new lights on the fundamental processes in life and introduced innovative methods to study structural and functional abnormalities in disease. It is satisfying to see that these excellent presentations are published in this monograph.

The holding of this symposium in Taiwan was most timely. There had already been a nucleus of scientists working on NMR. The gathering of the world's leading authorities provided a powerful magnet, and their superb lectures induced resonance among a broad spectrum of scientists and physicians in Taiwan. I am certain that the enthusiasm and excitement generated by this Symposium on Nuclear Magnetic Resonance will not decay with time, but rather this will usher in a new era of basic and clinical research in Taiwan. This symposium has provided the impetus for the scientists, physicians and the various institutions in Taiwan to begin a team effort to actively pursue this interdisciplinary approach and to make Taiwan an active contributor to this rapidly advancing frontier of biomedical research.

At this symposium, fertile seeds have been sown for the development of NMR research in biology and medicine. We will soon witness the blossoming of flowers and the bearing of fruits. I can envision that, in the near future, active biomedical studies on NMR will be conducted in Taiwan to probe the scientific truth of life and to improve the diagnosis and prevention of disease. These results will not only benefit the people in the Republic of China in Taiwan, but also contribute to the welfare and well–being of all mankind.

Subject Index

A

Acetic acid carboxylic proton image, 137–138

Acetic acid methyl proton image, 137–138

Acid-base perturbations, 211–214

Acidosis, 202

Acquisition time, 165

Acyl chain, 21

Adenine, 83, 84
  bond angle, 85, 86
  bond length, 85, 86
  x-ray crystallography, 84

Adenylate kinase, 5

ADP, 201, 218

Alamethicin, 66

Allosteric effector, 185

Alzheimer's disease, 165

Amino acid, ^{3}H-labeled, 28-30

Anemia, 159

Aneurysm
  dissecting aortic
    angiogram vs. magnetic resonance, 172, 173
  mycotic
    angiogram vs. magnetic resonance, 173, 174

Anisotropy, 10
  chemical shift, 34, 35
  fluorine, 8
  magnetic susceptibility, 59

Annulus fibrosus, vs. nucleus pulposus, 147–148

Aorta
  abdominal, 172
  arch, 168
  arteriosclerotic plaque, 175
    angiogram vs. magnetic resonance, 175, 176
  ascending, 167, 170
  descending, 168
  thoracic, 180

Artefact
  chemical shift, 138
  harmonics, 170
  interfacet, 149

Articular cartilage, disorders, 159–162

ATP, 185, 201, 218

synthesis, kinetic failure, 202

Atresia, tricuspid, 176, 177

Atrium
  left, 167, 171
  right, 170
  septal defect, 177

Auto-relaxation rate, 48

Axial image, 166

B

Back-projection, 136

Bacteriorhodopsin, 33–42
  anisotropic shift, 41
  isotropic shift, 41
  6-s-*trans* conformer, 41

Base-base stacking, 99–104

Beam-hardening effect, 141

Biochemistry, cellular, 217–238

Bond
  C = N, 38–40
  $C_{13} = C_{14}$, 37–38
  $C-4'-C-5'$, 91
  $C-^2H$, 21, 22
    orientational order parameter, 21
    rigid, 21
  NH-N, 108–110
  6-s, 40–41

Bone marrow, replacement disorders, 159

Brain
  arteriovenous malformation, 166, 167
  ^{31}P NMR, 230–231

Bronchus, 169

C

CAMELSPIN experiment, 52, 57, 62

Carbon, ^{13}C NMR, 113

Cardiac gating, 170
  arterial pulse, 170
  electrocardiogram, 167, 170, 179

Cardiac-respiratory gating, 168, 171–172

Cardiovascular system, 165–181

Carotid artery, 168, 180

Cartilage
  articular disorders, 159–162
  meniscal, 159–160

Cell membrane, protein-lipid interactions, 3–18

S

Sagittal image, 166
Scar tissue, 149
Schiff base
  ^{15}N, 34, 36–38, 40, 42
  protonated, 33, 37–40, 41–42
  unprotonated, 38, 41
Scintigraphy, radionuclide, 150
Sideband
  carbonyl, 35
  rotational, 34, 35
Signal intensity, 136
Signal-to-noise ratio, 138
Solid state technique, 33
Spatial resolution, 166
Spectroscopic reconstruction, three-
    dimensional, 137–138
Spectroscopy, zeugmatographic, 135
Spin, nuclear label, 19
Spin density, 142
spin echo technique, 138, 141-142
  hip, 153
  imaging sequence, 142, 144
Spin Hamiltonian, 8
Spin-spin splitting, 53, 58
Spinal cord, 143, 148
Spine, 146–149
  computed tomography, 146–149
  disease, 141
  fracture, 149
  stenosis, 149
  trauma, 163
Splitting
  quadrupole, 58
  spin-spin, 53, 58
Spondylolisthesis, 147
Stab wound, 176, 178
Stroke, 231
Subclavian artery, 168
Sugar ring
  envelope form, 91
  puckering, 91
  twist form, 91

T

Thalassemia, 160
Thecal sac, 143, 148
Thymine, 83, 84
  bond angle, 85, 86

bond length, 85, 86
  x-ray crystallography, 84
Tibia, 154–156
Tissue injury, 165
Tissue specificity, 165
Trachea, 169
Transfer function
  heart characteristics, 210, 211
  oxygen delivery regulation, 209–210
Trypsin inhibitor, bovine pancreatic, 19, 20
Tryptophan, 16
Tumor
  giant cell, 157–158
  lytic, femur, 157–158
  musculoskeletal, 153–158

U

Uracil, 83, 84
  bond angle, 85, 86
  bond length, 85, 86
  x-ray crystallography, 84

V

Valinomycin, 66
  dimyristoyl phosphatidylcholine, 67–76
  E. coli membrane model, 76–79
Valve, aortic, 170, 176, 177
Vascular disease, peripheral, 228–229
Vascular lumen narrowing, 180
Vascular system, 166–170
Vena cava, 172
  iliac branches, 172
  inferior, 169
  superior, 169
Ventricle
  left, 170
  septal defect, traumatic, 176, 178
Vinylphylloerythrin methyl ester, 59,
    60–62

W

Water proton image, 138

X

X-ray crystallography, 84, 93

Z

Zeugmatographic imaging, 135–140